Career or Fibromyalgia,

Do I Have to Choose?

Career or Fibromyalgia,

Do I Have to Choose?

The Practical Approach to Managing
Symptoms and the Life You Love

Karen R. Brinklow

NEW YORK

LONDON • NASHVILLE • MELBOURNE • VANCOUVER

Career or Fibromyalgia, Do I Have to Choose?

The Practical Approach to Managing Symptoms and the Life You Love

Published in New York, New York, by Morgan James Publishing in partnership with Difference Press. Morgan James is a trademark of Morgan James, LLC.
www.MorganJamesPublishing.com

ISBN 9781642798623 paperback
ISBN 9781642798630 eBook
ISBN 9781642798647 audiobook
Library of Congress Control Number: 2019953310

Cover & Interior Design by:
Christopher Kirk

Editor:
Bethany Davis

Book Coaching:
The Author Incubator

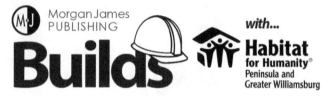

Morgan James is a proud partner of Habitat for Humanity Peninsula and Greater Williamsburg. Partners in building since 2006.

Get involved today! Visit
MorganJamesPublishing.com/giving-back

For Deanna and Dylan:
You've made being a mom the best job in the world.
I love you both around the world...and back again!

For Darrell:
Friendship is our foundation. Love is our precious gift.
It's pretty simple isn't it? Thank you for loving me!

For you:
When hope seems lost, never give up.

Table of Contents

Foreword

I first met Karen Brinklow in the fall of 2016 when she applied to join my Fibromyalgia Coach Training & Certification Program. Like many fibromyalgia patients, she was exhausted, in pain, and frustrated. Two years earlier, Karen had been forced to leave her dream career of being a teacher to go on medical leave. It broke her heart — and almost broke her. She reached out to me hoping to find a new purpose in life, helping others who were struggling with fibromyalgia. In her interview, Karen told me, "I need to feel vibrant and successful again. I used to absolutely love what I do but depression and fibromyalgia changed all of that. I want to feel joy again!" If you're reading this, I bet you can relate. Fibromyalgia can be a never-ending taking away of things. When left unmanaged, fibromyalgia slowly shrinks our lives to the point where we feel like a shadow or shell of who we used to be. Half of all fibromyalgia patients end up unable to work; one in five have filed some form of disability claim. Those who can work know their symptoms affect their productivity due to frequent absences, brain fog, pain, fatigue, and reduced work hours. We are also offered very little hope. Fibromyalgia patients are told: "There is no cure. Get used to your new normal." This is why Karen's story is so exciting! A few short years after her first conversation with me, Karen was able to go back to her dream career of teaching. In *Career or Fibromyalgia, Do I Have To Choose?,* Karen shares her story, as well as practical tips you can use on your journey. You will find a good healthy dose of hope within these pages! Most fibromyalgia patients have trouble even dreaming of what she actually accomplished. Her story proves that there are many things that can be done to help you feel better — even though there is no cure. In fact, your "new normal" can be just as fulfilling as your "old normal." Was it easy to bring her fibromyalgia and depression symptoms under control? I think Karen would be the first to tell you it wasn't! There was a lot of trial and error. She had to create her Dream Team of providers, including coaching, traditional medicine, and alternative therapies. There were many times that Karen was discouraged. When she had trouble holding on to hope and believing in a better future, those of us on her team would hope and believe for her. It took time to find the right treatment options and allow her body to heal. Karen also had to fight the medical system and advocate for herself to get the tests and treatments she needed. Most importantly, she learned to be gentler with herself, treating herself the way she would treat a cherished friend. Sometimes, Karen's hard work even looked like resting. Within these pages, you will find a very real and relatable story. I have no doubt that you will recognize yourself in the struggles Karen went through. My prayer is that you would also begin to see yourself in her success — and if you can't see it yet, know that Karen and I both believe for you. You can feel better than you do today! In chapter 3, Karen bluntly asks, "Is fibromyalgia a career killer?" I join Karen in emphatically saying, "No! It doesn't have to be!" If you are looking for ways to feel better and get back to a career you love, listen closely to what Karen has to say: she knows what she's talking about! Not only is she one of the finest coaches I've had the pleasure of training, but she's also "been there, done that" — and come back to thrive.

Tami Stackelhouse
Founder International Fibromyalgia Coaching Institute,
Bellevue, Washington
July 2019

Author's Note

*J*ust recently I've been joining private Facebook groups whose members all have fibromyalgia. When I was first realizing that fibromyalgia might be my secondary issue behind depression, I started looking everywhere for information and support. I came across these groups, but each time I tried to read through the posts I only felt worse. I was in denial that this was me. I didn't want to think that my life was going to only be pain, fatigue, and cognitive issues for the rest of my life. So, I didn't join any of those groups at the beginning of my journey.

When I signed on to write this book, I really thought it was going to centre around depression and supporting employees in the workplace, so their sick time was minimized. Nope!

It evolved to one about having to choose between fibromy-algia and the life and career you love. Now that it's written I have been curious about these Facebook groups again. It's not as difficult as it once was but it makes me so sad to hear of so many, many more than I ever thought, people suffering and that there looks to be little to no joy in their lives. This realization confirms that I have written the right book. I have lived their pain, frustration, and loss of hope. But I have also come out the other side of major depression and the struggle to manage fibromyalgia.

While I wanted to just give up many times, something inside me told me to press on because I knew I couldn't live like this the rest of my life. I didn't stop looking for answers. But this has been the hardest journey of my life. I believed I had no purpose anymore and felt hopeless. That inner voice kept pushing me forward even when I felt I couldn't any-more. After some grueling years I once again feel I have purpose in this life and have felt joy again in the job I love. But I also feel compelled to write this because I need to help others like me.

I now believe that going through this major challenge was and is still part of my life's purpose and the reason I have written this book. That inner voice is still pushing me and telling me the book is just the beginning. I have no idea where it will take me but am embracing that voice of guid-ance so that I fulfil my purpose. It's not up to me to choose that path but to follow my gut and help others.

I wrote this book for you! For me, it is the beginning of a new journey to help others find hope, happiness, and fulfillment in their lives once more. Joining those Facebook groups I mentioned has shown me how many people need that hope. I had no idea how many people are trying their best to cope with fibromyalgia and all that comes with it every day. I've been there and through determination and much trial and error I found a way to live life more purposefully.

Finding joy and purpose again might sound impossible to you right now. Trust me, it's not. I won't lie and tell you it's easy to get to, but I promise to be there with you so it won't take as long as it did for me. If you're serious about taking control of your fibromyalgia, keep reading. You are no longer alone and I can help you love life once again.

Thank you for purchasing this book. Now, let's start your journey back to living life the way you were meant to.

Chapter 1:

You're Not Alone

Myth: *Fibromyalgia is rare.*

Fact: *According to the National Fibromyalgia Association, ten million people in the United States and an estimated three to six percent of the world's population have fibromyalgia. In 2017 an estimated 500,000 Canadians are affected by fibromyalgia.*

*I*f you've picked up this book, good for you. You must be very frustrated. Maybe you're just about ready to give up on having a better quality of life and going back to the career you loved so much. But before you give up, I want to tell you the story of Nancy, a working professional just like you.

About ten years into her career, after switching her focus at work into a more demanding job, she began working at a pace and chronic stress level that she wasn't prepared for. She loved her job, so when the usual aches, pains, and tiredness that most people talk about started to be more of a problem she continued to push through. This is what she had always done to achieve her goals and, for the most part, it worked. But who doesn't push through while trying to raise a family and have a career at the same time? Plus, she also thought that maybe this is what aging feels like.

She was bringing home a lot of work and only taking one day on the weekend to spend with family and run errands. She started to wonder if this job was worth it all, but she loved it so much. She was finally in her dream career. Her children were beginning to notice how early she was going to bed and asking her if she was okay. She assured them she was fine. They also missed spending time together the way they did before she took on this new role. Then the pain started to increase and the fatigue/exhaustion set in. She began to go to bed earlier but continued to feel more and more exhausted.

About eight years into her career she switched into a more demanding role but she was confident in her ability to muscle through difficult times and come out the other side in a better place. Besides, she considered some of the stress to be positive stress that kept her moving forward and loving her job. However, Nancy did not see what was coming and how devastating it would be.

Like we all do, Nancy had a lot going on in her life. She had children, a fairly good marriage, could pay her bills, and tried her best to have a social life with family and friends. Nancy's family started to see subtle changes in her but didn't say anything. She was now exhausted coming home from work that used to make her energized even at the end of the day. She was often too tired to decide what to make for dinner and resorted to quick, easy meals that were not the healthiest but were easy to prepare and filled the hole. She stopped hosting family dinners as much because she was either too tired or had too much work on her plate that she had to bring home. She didn't know how to do the work in any way other than just to keep going. She didn't want to ask for help for fear of looking like a failure. This was not an option, so she continued at this pace.

Then things took a downturn and stresses were mounting in her job. Her work was piling up. She was now in survival mode. This began to take a toll on the rest of her life, but she was unaware of just how much it was affecting both her and her family. She began going to bed earlier and earlier. She started to need to sleep in more and would hit the snooze button several times, something she had never done in her life. Coffee, sweets, and carbs were fulfilling her cravings and she noticed she had put on some weight. She didn't worry about this because she was always able to keep this in check. She also didn't realize it was because of all her work stress. Nancy's overall pain in her body would ebb and flow, but was becoming more constant with each passing day. She was beginning to live for holidays so she could try and catch up on sleep. She felt like she had nothing to look forward to anymore and wondered if this was all worth it to have made a career change. She loved her job but was beginning to understand why some people became jaded and complained about their jobs. All Nancy wanted to do was feel better, because she *did* love her job. She felt like she was making a difference; she just wasn't sure she could continue this pace for the rest of her career. When her work tasks became more difficult and demanding, she started to get down on herself that she wasn't good at them, but what was she going to do? There was no way she was starting over again with something else, but she wasn't able to see clearly anymore to make decisions. She continued to press on.

Nancy tried to reach out to colleagues, but many were in the same boat and not opening up to talk about it. That just didn't happen – if it did, then you would really have to admit defeat. She was in more pain as well. But she had just ignored it, for the most part, and listened to others telling her to just push through, that it would be alright, it's what she needed to do, "It's what we all do." *Ugggh*, is that what having a career was?

Nancy's mood continued to decline and she was starting to run on autopilot and lose that sparkle that others used to comment on. She also started to notice times when she felt like blowing up or biting people's heads off. She knew at that point it was time to step back, but she didn't. She kept going at a pace that was going to take her down. The day came when she just couldn't do it anymore and she felt like crying most of the time. Nancy called her doctor and got an appointment to see her. After a few questions, Nancy's doctor told her she should not go back to work for a least a few weeks. Nancy's head started spinning, wondering what was going on. This kind of thing had never happened to her, but she knew she was just barely able to put one foot in front of the other at this point. So she relented and said okay, that she would take a few weeks. Her doctor prescribed her antidepressants and said to rest. Nancy didn't know what else to do now but go home.

A few weeks came and went and Nancy was feeling no better; in fact, her health was continuing to decline. As time went on, she became more and more frustrated, depressed, angry, and desperate to find answers, but she was too exhausted to be able to think straight and do the work she thought was necessary to be well again. As months went by, she was more and more dejected that the career she loved was over. She thought her working career in general was over, much less returning to the job she was so passionate about. She needed answers and a diagnosis but was getting nowhere other than her own obsession with researching online, trying desperately to figure out what was wrong with her. There must be an easy fix or more medication to set her on the right path, but what was it and where could she turn?

Nancy continued to read about many illnesses and could relate to them but continued to be more and more frustrated. One of the diagnoses she finally related to with all symptoms was fibromyalgia. It was time to ask her doctor about this.

If you're reading this book, your experience is likely much like Nancy's and you are not sure where to turn. This book is for you. In the chapters ahead I will tell you my story, which is much like Nancy's as well, and then I will show you how to manage symptoms and the life you love. I did it and you can too! I know you don't believe or feel that right now, but trust me and stay with me on this journey. I want to help you feel better, but I also want to help you get back to the job you love so much so that you can make the difference you were born to make.

Chapter 2:

My Story –
from Couch to Career

This is my story. It is very private and personal, but I feel that it is important to share because I don't want you to have to go through all the years it took me to get *me* back. While I was nervous about sharing such personal information and feelings the need to help others outweighed this. I want you to know that I have been there; I thought I would never be well, and I had lost all hope, especially of ever working again. While it took me years to find my job and passion for my job again, I'm making it my mission to help you get your spirit back and return to your career that ignites you.

I am a teacher. You may not be a teacher, but I know you're a driven professional who loves to succeed in things you're passionate about. It's who we are. But when that purpose and joy feels like it has been ripped away from you and is making you sick to the point that you feel your life is over and you will never work again – let alone feel joy – it's time to find someone who understands. That's why I am writing this for you. I want you to have someone who understands, who's been there and is dedicated to taking the journey with you to once again feel passion and joy so you can return to the dream job you cared so much about. This is why I am wearing my heart on my sleeve and sharing my personal journey so that you don't have to take years to begin to feel better.

From the time I was eight years old, I knew I wanted to teach. I used to set up desks in my basement and put stuffed animals in them while I pretended to be the teacher at the front of the class. As a teenager I taught Sunday school, piano lessons, and summer day camps. But my dream didn't quite get there when it should have. At thirty-seven, a brief window of opportunity opened that gave me hope of becoming a teacher again. As a family, we decided I would go for it. At thirty-seven, I was accepted into a university within an hour's drive from my home. This in itself was an accomplishment and I felt so lucky and blessed to be moving toward my goal of becoming a teacher. At the time, my children were thirteen and eleven. We all made a conscious decision to give up our annual ski trips so that I could go after my dreams. The bank said they would only lend us $10,000 for me to go. That only covered part of the first year, including all of my living expenses and the expenses of going to and from school. We believed that I was meant to do this and that the money to do so would come. It did, each year the bank approved more money. While I was going to have loans that needed to be paid back, I knew that it was an investment in me and the payoff would come in a job.

I was thriving at university and loved what I was learning. I had to complete my undergrad before I could apply to do my Education degree. There was no guarantee I would be accepted into their education program after undergrad, but I was told by the dean that if I kept my marks high I had a chance. Three years later I was attending the Faculty of Education and my dream of becoming a teacher was within reach!

Unfortunately, jobs were scarce when I graduated and even though I had a great resume from my working years, had graduated with distinction, and received an award, I did not get a full-time job. You see, getting a teaching job is a little more political than I ever thought. I came from a place where if you work hard and set and reach goals, then you are rewarded. This political stuff was new for me and quite honestly I didn't get it because it didn't seem right to me. But I persisted and after three years was hired to my dream job! I will never forget that day and how I felt. It was overwhelming and exhilarating to make it. I was flying high and felt like my struggles and hard work had finally paid off and I would have the job security that I was so looking for. I wanted to provide significantly more financially for my family, help my children with university, and provide for my own retirement. This was a great financial plan in my mind. I just didn't see the roadblock I was about to hit with full force coming, the one that would knock me down for four and a half years.

A few years into teaching, I was beginning to feel confident and get a handle on all the preparation and planning of new courses that is quite challenging at the beginning of a teaching career. This was exhausting and stressful, but I knew there was a light at the end of the tunnel when I would be able to repeat teaching some courses in the future. This light was within reach when things beyond my control dropped a boulder in my path that set into motion a chain of events that left me with chronic illnesses I will need to manage for the rest of my life. Amidst all of this, my marriage ended and added to the mountain of challenges I was about to face.

As time went on, I was not the same person. Like Nancy – and I am sure you – I was exhausted, in pain all over, and my thinking was foggy. Coffee was my go-to for energy and to help clear the fuzziness. As I said, there had been circumstances beyond my control that forced me to teach too many new courses in too many schools in too short of a timeframe. I kept rising to the challenge and was determined to ride this horrible storm out and come out the other side all the better for it. But the opposite started to happen. I was getting worse without realizing the negative effects it was having on me. Then one day, in the fall of 2013, I couldn't do it anymore. I called my doctor, went to see him, and he took me off work immediately due to stress. This only made me feel worse. There is such a negative stigma around having to take sick leave for stress that I felt like a failure and just wanted to hide. That is exactly what I did. I stayed on my couch and slept most of the day. My doctor had put me on antidepressants and said that I needed to rest. I knew my doctor was treating me for depression, but we never really talked about a label as such. We talked about the symptoms I had and how much time I needed off work. That time just kept getting longer and longer.

I was in so much pain, physically and mentally exhausted, and knew that I needed to take some time off but felt like a failure because I couldn't keep going. I had also come to hate my job and this devastated me because I had loved it so much and because for so long it had been my dream. It only took a short time to take that from me. I was angry, bitter and depressed, in pain, exhausted, and couldn't think straight.

My few weeks off turned into a few months. Things only continued to get worse with my health, and I was still off work. I continued to not feel better. I was seeing my doctor every two months and he continued to keep me off work. I was only existing and not living, and losing hope as time continued to pass. The medication didn't seem to be working, as I was not getting better. My symptoms were all over the place and when I felt better one day, the next I would feel worse. I read too much and continued to confuse myself even more. My brain had cognitive issues that didn't allow me to organize information to make sense. It just felt like a huge burden to try and make sense of things, and I didn't have the energy to focus on anything, much less on managing my symptoms. I was living the worst part of it alone and not sharing much with anyone. I kept the severity of how I felt to myself. I thought by thinking positively that maybe, just maybe, I could feel better. However, that was not the case.

I had lost all hope of ever working again, let alone having the passion to teach. I could not see that was even an option for me. I became obsessed with researching my symptoms and chasing jobs. I still believed I should be working and if I could only prove myself with another perceived successful career, I would be better. I now believe God had other plans for me. Stay with me here, please. This book is not a preachy or religious book, but I have to give credit where credit is due, at least how I see it. I believe writing this book is part of that plan so that I can help others.

My symptoms are much like yours, if not the same, and I want to help you more than you know. I continued to obsess over my symptoms and search for jobs online. After a few interviews, I finally gave up, because even if I was the successful candidate, I knew in my heart I couldn't do the jobs because of my health and I was still devastated I couldn't teach. Besides, all my symptoms were still there. Did I believe that magically they would disappear if I could just prove I was successful again? Yup, I did.

I was on a rollercoaster of emotions and essentially hiding from people and my former life in education. I was managing depression and anxiety and angry at life for handing me this curveball. I had faced many challenges up to this point, but this one felt like a sledgehammer had hit me in the stomach. I knew I did not have the energy or wellness to be able to pursue another career or take any more education to change course again. The hardest part of all was that I had worked so hard at getting my degree and my teaching certification that I felt like all my dreams had been ripped from me.

A few months into my sick leave, I decided to make an appointment with a naturopathic doctor. I had heard of someone who was really good in the small town near me. In winter of 2014, I began seeing her and following a regimen with food changes, no gluten, dairy, or eggs. She also had me on meal replacement shakes for extra nutritional support in addition to supplements. The biggest change for me then was weight loss. This was awesome, because I knew I could stand to lose about fifteen to twenty pounds. I really thought this was going to be my "magic pill," but I gradually stopped going. I was still exhausted and depressed. I had lost the weight though, so that was good.

I chased many other treatments. As I'm writing this, I realize the circles I ran around in trying to find answers to help me. I was still hoping there was a magic pill, but the more things I read about and tried, the more I began to realize what a difficult journey I was going to need to take to have my dream back. Keep in mind that the entire time I was doing all of this, I still thought my issue was stress – whatever that meant – from work and all I needed were rest and relaxation, and medication to help with depression.

In spring of 2014, my short-term sick leave ran out, I was still no better and my doctor said no to my going back to work. I didn't argue, because I knew I couldn't do my job. I knew I couldn't do *any* job, for that matter. I really thought my career might be over and it made me both sad and angry. Why did this have to happen to me? I now needed to apply for long-term disability through my insurance company at work.

You may experience this challenge with sick leave, too; you may have to apply for long-term disability or a government disability plan after you've exhausted your short-term plan. This can be a rigorous and time-consuming process and it requires a lot of thinking. No wonder so many people give up and don't apply! Don't put this off. By the time you get to this point, your mental state may be having difficulty processing having to do this. I did not want to do this, and it has to do with the stigma you hear from people not understanding why it's important to have this benefit or judging you for needing to do it. All of this does not help you. I was reluctant to tell anyone, so we didn't. This was also contributing to the stigma. I was stressed about having to apply. I had no choice, though. I still had bills to pay. After taking the time and putting as much thought into this application as I could, I was easily approved and would be able to be off now for up to two years if necessary.

There was a significant drop in our household income due to this change, but somehow, we managed. I was budgeting and keeping spending to a minimum. Plus, I did not have the energy to go anywhere, let alone into a store to shop, which I don't like to do anyway!

Some positive things were happening in my life, and in the summer of 2014 I married the best man I have ever known. I was the happiest I had been in a long time and this really helped me to once again feel that maybe I was on the road to getting better. I thought that by focusing on being the best wife I could be, I could be fulfilled at never working again. My husband was very supportive and loved having me home. While this was an awesome feeling, it also made me feel more pressure to succeed at being a house-wife, which only added to my diminishing health. Doing all the things necessary to run a successful household required energy that I just didn't have. It took me a while to be able to let go of that, as it did make me feel like a failure once again.

I had massages during this time, but they were infrequent at best, as I was still waiting for my antidepressants and rest-ing to work. I only went every few months or so, when I felt really bad. Massage exhausted me and I had to go home and rest after. I tried acupuncture, which was entirely new for me. I was skeptical but trusted my massage therapist and her credentials, so when she recommended acupuncture I thought, "Why not?" Like massage, it helped in the short term. I eventually just gave up on this too.

Showering, getting dressed, and doing my hair were exhausting and turned into a three-step process. I couldn't shower every day because of the fatigue. It was just too much. The days I did, I needed to lie down after shower-ing just to get the energy to get dressed. Often, after I got dressed, I would rest again before doing my hair. Holding the hairdryer was tiring as well. Something so simple that we take for granted had become a chore. Standing to do this was exhausting and my husband searched to find me a dressing table so I could sit to do my hair and makeup. This was so helpful. He continues to look for ways to support me and help me do things more efficiently. To this day I still use my dressing table and it is only on very rare occasions now that I need to rest in between showering and getting dressed and doing my hair.

I decided to look into more treatment options and that led me to yoga and meditation. I had read lots in my research about yoga being helpful for fibromyalgia, so I found a yoga studio and signed up for that. I loved yoga and it made my body feel so good. It was exhausting, but it really helped to calm down the pain in my muscles. But then winter hit and I stopped going so much for many reasons – weather, cold, and I didn't want to go out of the house after dark. There was always a good reason not to go. During my yoga phase, I also tried meditation and signed up for a six-week class for this. I enjoyed it, but I'm not sure how much it helped at that time. It was a good practice to help me relax and let go of stresses in my life, but I found it hard to make this a consistent practice of daily living. I was still so exhausted all the time and it would tire me out even more. Depression also zaps motivation, which is something I will be dealing with the rest of my life as well.

In the spring of 2015, my husband and I flew to China to visit my daughter. This was an amazing opportunity as she decided to work abroad for a year. It was also way less expensive than we thought it would be. We also thought it would be a restful vacation for me to have and might help to get my health moving in the right direction. I was still taking the medications my doctor had prescribed. He had made several adjustments by now because my mood was still quite low, along with fatigue, pain, and brain fog. We had to do a lot of walking in China and even though this was exhausting, I thought it was the right thing to be doing to help my body so I continued to push myself. I still didn't know at this point that I was also dealing with fibromyalgia and the amount of walking I was doing was not good for me.

In summer of 2015 we sold our home and bought another one. Thankfully it sold quickly, I was concerned about how we would keep it ready to show because I knew I couldn't keep up with that. We wanted to move to a country setting and have a place big enough to accommodate my aging parents. We found the perfect house, but having to get ready to move was extremely difficult for me. I paced myself and would pack a bit and then rest. This was so hard, and I couldn't keep up with how much there was to do. I did not ask anyone for help because it only made me feel like a failure to have to admit I needed the support. A month before Christmas, we moved into our new home, but even on moving day we still had stuff to pack. Organizing a new house after a move was more than I could handle. I had to be satisfied with it not being perfect, not even close. A month after we moved in, my daughter surprised us and showed up to help my parents move in and settle. What a godsend she was! She could see how exhausted and tired I was all the time, too. It was certainly more difficult to not let people see how sick I was, because there were others in the house now during the day when I was used to spending that time alone. Even though I did my best to not show how ill I was, I know my husband could see it. He never really said too much, but I know he worried a lot. After my parents moved in they also saw how sick I was and this worried me because I knew they were worried about me.

At one of my family doctor follow-ups, I asked him if I might have fibromyalgia. I had eliminated many other things on my own from researching them and asking him about them. I had been doing a lot of research on depression, pain, and fatigue, which also led me in the direction of fibromyalgia. This didn't help, because there are stigmas around both depression and fibromyalgia and talking to people about them only made me feel like I was more of a failure. I'm sure my doctor was ready to throttle me at this point, but he was patient. When I asked about fibromyalgia, he said it was unlikely I had it because I did not have pressure points that were painful, a common symptom. I had all the other symptoms and had determined myself that I actually did have these pressure points. I knew this from having massage treatments. He checked me and, yes, he confirmed it then. He said that I was taking the best meds to help fibromyalgia – antidepressants. This left me feeling even worse, especially when I had been reading and learning all about fibromyalgia on my own. I had been thinking, "If I could just get an answer, then we could treat it." I thought my fibromyalgia diagnosis was my magic answer.

I asked the doctor if he was going to refer me to a rheumatologist, because that was something else I had read about. He said no, that they were not seeing fibromyalgia patients anymore as there was nothing they could do for them. So I was still at square one. As you may know by now on your own journey, fibromyalgia is not easy to diagnose. It looks different on different people and it does not have a lot of support in the medical field. This, however, is changing, albeit slowly.

My quest for help didn't stop and I was searching more now online and reading everything I could get my hands on about fibromyalgia. The more I searched and read, the more confused I was about how to manage my health. I was beginning to think there might not be a magic pill for this after all and that my journey was going to be a difficult one. I was learning a lot on my own but getting nowhere with my own health, so I kept googling. I cried a lot when I was alone too, I was grieving the loss of myself and my career.

In the spring of 2016, my initial long-term disability changed definition from "own occupation" to "any occupation." I received devastating news that the insurance company I paid into at work did not approve any more long-term disability. They thought I could do *any* job. This made me feel terrible about myself. I was angry and frustrated with this. It only worsened my symptoms. I told them that if I could do any job, I would be teaching. My doctors were stunned. This was a horrible time, as I didn't know what we would do without any income from me. I knew I couldn't work, and my doctor confirmed this. This only added to my stress and increased the pain and the symptoms of depression and anxiety. Despite the lengthy letters and application from myself and my doctors, explaining how I was living day-to-day, they felt fibromyalgia would be fixed by doing some light exercise like walking. No lie! What a slap in the face. They didn't have to live the way I was. I then was forced to apply for government pension disability. This was even less money coming in and stressed me out even more. This was crazy because I was really sick and my insurance company that I had paid into for so long had let me down. At this point they ignored the depression diagnosis and just decided fibromyalgia was not a real illness. I kid you not! They were horrible to me.

When I applied for my government disability, though, what a difference. I was treated like a human being and they were compassionate. I was approved! The crazy thing was that, to be approved for government disability, I had actually submitted the exact same application and documentation that my insurance company had denied. With some creative budgeting I knew it was enough to contribute and make ends meet.

Finally, I got to the point where I could not keep going on feeling like this. I was never suicidal, but I did think about death and that is what scared me. In the summer of 2016, I was truly at my very worst. I was tired of the "hamster wheel" approach, hoping something would stick. The depressed mood I was experiencing was really low. By now, I'm sure you know how much effort it takes to just get dressed to go do anything and how you have to paste a smile on your face and pretend you're okay. Pretending was much easier than having to exhaust myself trying to explain something that was complex even for me to understand after so much research (and now, education), let alone someone who had lots of questions and no knowledge – or partial knowledge – of the problem.

At the next check-in with my doctor, I said, "I can't take this anymore." He wanted to make yet another medication change and I said no, I wanted a referral to a psychiatrist for drug-resistant depression. He agreed and sent the referral. I needed help and I knew the expertise a psychiatrist has with medication, so it felt like the logical next step. I knew I couldn't live like this the rest of my life and there had to be a better way and solutions to improve my health. I guess I was stubborn, because I didn't give up with searching for hope and help.

I was lucky enough to get a call from the psychiatrist's office and was scheduled to see her in a few months. The depression I had was hitting rock bottom and I was counting the days to see the psychiatrist. While waiting to see her, I did more research on fibromyalgia. This was daunting because there is way too much information out there to process (fibro brain) and there are so many schools of thought that I just felt more frustrated about how I was ever going to get better. If you've been diagnosed, you know what I'm talking about and you're ready to get someone to help you through. If not, don't be alarmed, because I've been through a journey that will allow me to be there for you and get you going on a path to feeling better.

I am a researcher and curious by nature. I love learning and getting the facts, and university taught me how to think and to analyse information for credibility. The real fact is that getting answers on fibromyalgia is tough because there's much stuff out there and everyone seems to have an opinion on everything. One such opinion that really made me feel bad was someone saying, "Oh, that's just a catch-all diagnosis when doctors don't know what's wrong with you," and also, "That's just the new fad illness." These comments didn't help and only made me feel stupid and more inclined to keep everything to myself. It wasn't until I had done all my research that I realized this is a very real illness. Doctors are trained to give you a pill to make the symptoms go away. Fibromyalgia doesn't work that way, so it's no wonder they find it frustrating to deal with patients who have it.

During my fibromyalgia research I came across someone whose story sounded just like mine! Probably the same way you've found me – I was desperately searching for help and answers. So I reached out to her. I told myself she might be the one to give me a magic pill and tell me I was going to be alright. When Tami called me back, I was at my worst. I'm sure I sounded desperate to her and I know I cried – a lot – with her on the phone. Thank God she was such a caring human being. She made me feel listened to and could speak from her own experience with fibromyalgia, so I believed what she was telling me because it sounded just like me. She also validated me being sick. This felt like a weight off my shoulders at the time. At this point she was the only solution I thought held some hope for me and was the only person who had the best, most comprehensive knowledge that I had found. She was also a fibromyalgia coach. I had no clue what that was, but she was so understanding that I felt like I was being cared for by a best friend.

I was considering investing in and working with her to help me sort out my health when she told me she thought she had a better solution for me. She had just started training others to coach people with fibromyalgia to lead better lives. So this is where I invested, in becoming a fibromyalgia advisor. Still thinking my teaching career was over, I saw this as a possible new career path. I could look after myself, help others, and convince myself I was still teaching. I learned so much about fibromyalgia and won an award for excellence. I was ready to take on the world again, or so I thought. The more I looked at building a business coaching others, the more I realized how long it was going to take, and I had already spent years going to university doing that to have a teaching career. The biggest factor, though, was I still wasn't well enough to take on this endeavour. If I could have, I would have been back in the classroom. This was another devastating blow emotionally, and my hope faded again. By now, you may have tears in your eyes the way I did when I began to read through Tami's experience and how much like mine it was. I know you're hurting and don't know where to turn, but stay with me as I show you there is a better place to be than where you are now.

During the time I was taking the advisor course, I began seeing my new psychiatrist. She was amazing and, like Tami, made me feel validated and understood. I truly believe she saved my life. I was at rock bottom when I finally got to my appointment with her. I will never forget her taking hold of my hands and promising I was going to feel better. She couldn't promise when, but she did promise to stick with me until I did, however long that took. She diagnosed me with major depression and generalized anxiety disorder and supported the fibromyalgia diagnosis. She made major changes to the medications I was already on and asked me to trust her when I felt reluctant to add more medications. She explained that it might take many medication tweaks and changes, and I needed to provide feedback on side effects if I had them in order to get just the right ones for me. The next thing she needed to address was my fatigue. Luckily, she was also a sleep specialist and ordered me to go for a sleep study. I was being monitored very closely by this doctor and I now know I was more sick than I realized. But admitting that was quite another thing. I only shared this with my husband. He knew more than I that I was in a bad state. I cannot express my gratitude and love for him enough for the support, love, and friendship that we share. If not for his support, I'm not sure where I would be today.

The sleep study revealed sleep apnea. What?! Even the sleep education leader was surprised because I do not look like a candidate for sleep apnea. Side note, I never looked like I was depressed and I never looked like I had fibromyalgia either. Remember, these are invisible illnesses that you cannot see! Not to mention that I didn't let most people see them, either. Who wants to go out looking bad?! Ah, no one, so why would I go out looking like I had depression and fibromyalgia? Anyway, because of the sleep apnea diagnosis I was scheduled to try a continuous positive airway pressure (CPAP) machine. I did not want to, but I knew I needed to in order to try and find help, especially with the fatigue. I even heard comments around sleep apnea being another fad diagnosis. I'm sure you can guess how this made me feel.

About nine months into seeing the psychiatrist, I was getting frustrated because I was not feeling any change in the depression. I was still struggling with pain and fatigue and was trying to implement strategies to help the fibromyalgia from the advisor course I had taken. This was somewhat helpful, but because of the depression I was still on a hamster wheel of symptoms. I wasn't even sure the CPAP machine was beneficial, but according to the doctor it was improving my sleep somewhat. I was beginning to be resistant to all the medication tweaks and changes the psychiatrist was suggesting, as some were making me feel sick. But I persevered because I felt I was in good hands. After yet another medication adjustment in July, 2017, I felt something different. It was a tiny feeling, but I knew something had changed and was changing in my mood. This was the beginning I needed to feel. I was scared to believe it or acknowledge it for fear it was not really happening. This was the part that had to happen before I could begin to address the fibromyalgia symptoms and have some significant progress. I began to implement small, manageable strategies from what I learned about fibromyalgia and my psychiatrist asked me to take part in psychodynamic therapy. I also had symptoms of PTSD, and she said this talk therapy would help to address any underlying issues that I was unaware of that were holding me in a state of depression. Once again, I trusted her and said I would try anything as I was starting to feel a change. I began attending the sessions on a weekly basis and would continue with that for one year. That seemed like forever, but I didn't have a choice because I wanted to move forward with my health.

After a couple of months of the new medication and attending the counselling, I told my psychiatrist that I was actually thinking about work and teaching again. I couldn't believe that those feelings were in me and it surprised me where they were coming from. She did not want me to move too quickly with these things and said okay, that we could think about it. This was in September 2017, and school had just begun. I love September and seeing the busses and hearing the excited students at the beginning of the year. But I was also sad because I was not part of it. However, for the first time in four years I had hope and a feeling that maybe I wanted to try to work my way back. When my doctor was ready to let me try, she would only let me return slowly and gradually. In December of that same year, I started by volunteering at a couple of one-hour classes a week until the next semester started. In February of 2017, I started teaching again, but I only had my doctor's permission to try teaching one class. This was a milestone moment and it was difficult, as it caused my symptoms to flare again. I had accomplished so much by now that this felt like starting over again as the daily exhaustion and pain became worse again. I had to learn to manage these symptoms while working without ending up back where I once was. My psychiatrist had been really strict about my return to work and had not allowed me to take things too quickly. That had been a challenge to overcome because I started to feel like maybe I could handle full time. Deep down I knew I couldn't, but I was making baby step progress, and more than anything I had hope again for a teaching career. As you know, even baby steps for someone like you and me is a huge challenge and takes time to embrace. Strangely enough, once you do, you begin to make improvements more quickly. I often think about the tortoise and the hare story when I get frustrated with how long it's taking me to recover from flares.

The next major step forward was in September of 2018, when I added another course to my teaching timetable. Mornings are still difficult for me, but we accommodated that by making my timetable only afternoon classes. This was working. It was another slight step back to adjust to the increase, but with strategies in place and a consciousness of what my body was telling me, since then I have been able to make continuous improvements and manage my overall symptoms. When I say "continuous improvements," it does not mean that I am better. It means that I am able to reduce symptoms and manage them so I can work and do more of the things I love.

Another big step forward at this time was in the therapy sessions. I was feeling I didn't need them anymore. Without much awareness, things were changing from these sessions and I had come to a point where I knew I was ready to move forward from them.

These days, my life is looking good. I love my teaching career again. My goal was to increase to full time midway through second semester, but that had to be put off until the next school year begins. I know this is the right decision because my gut told me not to go too fast and to give myself the time I need to prepare my body for full-time work, if that is possible. I am also writing this book for you and never in my wildest dreams did I think I would be where I am. While I still work and strategize to manage my health on a daily, weekly, and monthly basis, I am on a good path to feeling joy and fulfillment once again. This book is for you. Let me walk this path with you (because we don't run anymore) so that you can find your hope and joy. I know you can do it. If I can, you can and I will be with you all the way. Now let me tell you about the journey I can take you on so you can get back to the career you love!

Chapter 3:

Let Me Take You on a Journey

*Myth: Nothing can be done for fibromyalgia. You
just have to learn to live with the pain.*

Fact: *Although there is not yet a cure for
fibromyalgia, it can be managed with the right
combination of treatments, therapies, and support.*

The following journey I want to share with you is the
one that finally allowed me to get unstuck and begin
to find relief so that I could find hope, wellness, and
joy again. I don't want you to have to do this alone or take
years like I did to get back to my dream job. Is fibromyal-

gia a career killer? I sure thought so, and thought I would never be able to work again. At the end of this book I want you to be able to answer that question with an emphatic *no* and make the decision to take complete charge of your life and get back to the work that brings you joy and happiness. The path that I took that finally got me back to the job I love was too long. You will be able to see how I did it and you can, too. I have no doubt. I need you to be open to anything to help you. It's easy to find excuses about what won't work and why you won't try something, but that thinking will keep you stuck. What works for some doesn't work for others, and I got stuck listening to too much stuff and to people thinking they knew what was wrong with me. I had to start listening to my body and in particular to my gut. I taught my kids to always follow their gut as it will never steer you wrong. I still believe it to this day and I now teach students this strategy and how to listen to your gut to guide you. I also had to stop listening to the stigma around depression and medications and be able to share my experience so that others don't have to feel alone and can feel better. There are still many who don't know my journey, as it's still difficult to share. This book is giving me the platform to share and especially to help you.

It's easy to be taken off course, especially when you are sick and feeling no hope. You can continue to decline and then have a bigger hill to climb to feel better. I was always the person who came into work or entered a room happy, joyful, and full of hope. People often teased me about it. I missed being that person and am still working on getting that completely back. Depression killed that in me, at least for a while. Those negative thoughts that depression keeps in the back of your mind are really hard to stop listening to so you can fulfil your life's purpose. While I continue to manage that and the symptoms of fibromyalgia, I am on my way to a place I never thought would be possible. I want to help you get there too and in a much shorter time than it took me. "The Practical Approach" will help you to narrow your focus and sort out all that information so that you feel less overwhelmed and more in control. While it's okay to choose where to start acting upon my tips, I suggest that before you do, you read each chapter in order. I have written it in the order that got me to where I am today. I just didn't have a plan in front of me to follow. I want you to stop feeling so frustrated and searching online for hours for solutions. I want to help you get out of the cycle of confusion and help you to feel some of the pressure has lifted off of your shoulders. I want you to see the light at the end of the tunnel and feel that it is getting bigger and closer for you. I want to see your pain and fatigue get some relief so you can begin to feel focused and organized again. I want you to be able to manage your symptoms so that you have a plan to get back to the career you love!

In the chapters I will help you answer the following questions:

- How did I get here?
- What's wrong with me?
- What can I do to feel less alone?
- How do I get stuff done and focus on being well?

- What are my treatment options?
- How will I know I'm starting to improve?
- Am I really thinking I can work again?
- Why am I having a bad day again?

In my personal chapter, "My Story – From Couch to Career," I helped you to see that you are not alone by sharing my journey with you. By doing this, I hope you see that you too can get to a point where you love your life again and consider going back to a job you love.

In the chapter "How Did I get Here?" I will help you reflect on your life and begin to see what led to the decline of your health. Sometimes we can pinpoint the exact time this happened and sometimes it's a culmination of things over time. There was a combination of both that caused me to get sick. I did not realize it was happening to me until it was too late. I'm willing to bet this is true for you as well.

In "It's All in My Head" I discuss the many real symptoms that you may have and are not sure what to do or where to turn. You will begin to understand your symptoms so that you can start your journey to improvement.

In "Why Do I Feel So Alone?" I help you to understand why you have these feelings and how to acknowledge them so you can move forward toward positive change and improvements.

In "How Do I Get Stuff Done and Focus on Being Well?" I offer you some tips and tricks that I used to be able to balance illness and getting things done that still needed attention, all while trying to make little bits of progress. While this might seem impossible, it just takes some creative thinking to find solutions to help you. Once you can do this, you will be able to feel more positively about your situation and focus on what matters most to your improvements and managing your symptoms.

In "Treatments: Traditional, Alternative, or Both?" I offer ideas for you to consider that I tried, and those that worked and continue to do so. It really is a balancing act that takes some time to work through, but when things begin to improve you will feel much better about trying different approaches that will work for you.

I think that, "Am I Really Starting to Feel Better?" is my favourite chapter, because this is where I learned through trial and error things that worked for me and continue to do so. Once I started to realize I needed to take a slower, more methodical approach to seeing what would work, I then started to see little improvements. That started the ball rolling toward having many more good days than bad.

In "Wow! I Think I'm Ready to Work Again!" I share my path back to work and all the strategies I needed in order to follow that path. While you may not think this is possible right now, trust me, it is and I am with you all the way.

Finally in "Why Am I Having a Bad Day Again?" I address how and why you may have a bad day after you start to feel more improvements and begin to add more back into your life. You will see that the bad days will be fewer and fewer and that when you do have one you know what to do to recover quickly. You will learn the importance of self-care and how having someone in your corner to support you on your own journey will help you to get there faster.

It is possible to feel joy again! It is possible to get back to your job again! It is possible to feel empowered to take control of your symptoms so that you can feel your best again. Allow me to take this road with you. I will be there when it gets rough and bumpy and you feel like giving up, and I will be there in the end to help you celebrate your successes as you find joy, happiness, and purpose once more. Just turn the page and take it one baby step at a time. I am with you.

Chapter 4:

How Did I Get Here?

Myth: *Fibromyalgia is a "wastebasket diagnosis" doctors use when they can't figure out what's wrong with you.*

Fact: *There is a specific set of diagnostic criteria used for diagnosing fibromyalgia. It takes time to get to the diagnosis because so many other things need to be ruled out.*

F ibromyalgia sucks! Any chronic illness sucks for that matter, but fibromyalgia is so misunderstood and mysterious. Right now you're likely saying, why me?

What the heck did I do to deserve this? You finally got your dream job (or one you love) and then *BOOM*, it's like you're taken out by the "linebacker" of fibromyalgia.

So where did it all begin? How can you possibly figure it out when you are exhausted, in pain, and your brain seems to be in a constant fog? You are also probably thinking, "I need answers!"

Understanding what led you to getting sick isn't easy, *but* when you start reflecting and paying attention to what may have led to this point you will be surprised how easy those answers will come.

Wrapping your head around the symptoms associated with fibromyalgia and depression is hard. My thoughts were conflicted because I assumed that successful people who have always gotten through tough times don't take sick leave. I really believed this to be a weakness on my part. This did not help me one bit. I am a resourceful person and always researching because I am curious by nature. I love learning! But understanding and admitting to what led to my getting sick was tough. That's why I want to help you and simplify what took me so long to figure out. I know you're needing simple steps and answers because you're too exhausted and your brain just can't handle the kind of thinking needed right now to do what you want to do – research. On the other hand, I know you're googling like crazy looking for answers and getting more and more confused and stressed.

My two biggest fears were "What will people think?" and "I can't afford to be sick!" I'm positive you're thinking this because that's what people like you and me think first, "What will people think?" I want to you stop right now and consider something. Does it matter what people think? What people are you worried about the most? Are the people you're worried about the ones you should be giving thinking time to? Not in the least! The people who matter most will only care about you, first and foremost. If that is just one person, then so be it, and if that person is me, I am so happy you decided to pick up this book. I am here for you and I understand.

Let's talk about going on sick leave. I know as well as you do that it's there for a reason. But you rarely use it, correct? The reason it's there is for times like these, and yes, it's okay to take the time the doctor has told you to take because you're so stressed out that he thinks it's time for a rest. Ask yourself this: can I *really* not afford it? For a short time anyway, you can and you should.

Racking your brain on a daily basis is exhausting in itself. Beating yourself up is exhausting and leads to more exhaustion, stress, and negative thinking, which only makes you feel worse. But how the heck do you get off this hamster wheel and find focus again?

It's time to begin to understand why you are here now. You may not be able to pinpoint exactly why, but with thoughtful reflection I'm betting you can figure out that source. Once you begin to understand why you got to this horrible place, then you will be able to get the answers you need.

Stress! Take a moment to sit back and self-reflect. Can you see that stress is a huge factor at this point? I never thought for a minute that stress would lead me to having a chronic illness, let alone fibromyalgia. Like you, I had always come through many stressful times, as bad as they were, relatively unscathed. I prided myself that I could handle stress and recover from tough times. I was nowhere close to handling the stress that knocked me down and stripped me of my identity and sense of purpose.

Looking at your reflection, can you see that over time you continued to up the ante and meet every challenge placed upon you? You thrived on those challenges and it's what drove you to be successful and fulfilled, right? Then why, from out of nowhere, did your doctor say you need a break from work?

I know you love your career. I know how devastated you are to be on sick leave, but you need to begin to understand what led to you getting sick.

Were you:

- Burning the midnight oil
- Trying to be all things to all people
- Saying yes to whatever was asked of you at work
- Striving for perfection
- Being the best wife, mother, and employee possible
- On a steep learning curve in your career for too long with no end in sight
- Keeping all the stress to yourself, pasting a smile on your face, and pretending to be the perfect employee while everyone around you was successful and looked like they were not stressed
- Putting too much pressure on yourself to be the best

- Not taking the time on weekends to let work go and focus on you and your family
- Letting yourself be last
- Not exercising
- Stress eating – especially breads, chips, chocolate, and other sweets
- Stressed because you couldn't keep up with house-work and your job and feeling guilty because of it
- Not sleeping well – couldn't get to sleep, couldn't stay asleep, woke up several times in the night or early in the morning
- Struggling to put one foot in front of the other and feeling guilty when someone told you just to keep pushing through because that's what they do?

I could go on and on, but I think that is more than enough to start your reflection on what led you to be here. Not just stress, but massive amounts of accumulating chronic stress that you didn't see because you are an achiever, a go-get-ter, and nothing stops you…right? Until *bam*! You have no choice but to go on sick leave and take some time to get better and back to the job you love. You can afford sick leave.

At this point, I hope you have started to have some idea of what led you to getting sick. If not, no worries, as focusing on that too long can keep you in a negative space where you can't focus on being well. Now that you have an idea of what led you to getting sick, next let's look at loss of purpose. For me, this was devastating. More so, I was embarrassed. Embarrassed? I was sick but my pride kept me focused on what people think, embarrassed I could not keep up, and that led to a profound sense of loss of purpose. I can't say this enough, it was devastating and I'm sure you're beyond devastated to be where you are.

Lying on the couch day in and day out, frantically searching the internet for answers only left me more confused and traumatized. Exhaustion kept me on the couch but gave me too much time to search for answers. Then I would sleep. I would shower before my husband came home from work and then prepare dinner. It was all I could do while trying to pretend I had been busier all day. I was home and should be able to manage the household. After all, I wasn't working, so I should be productive at home. But I didn't grasp the significance of why my doctor had taken me off work. I knew I needed answers.

I like to research and get answers and make good decisions based on solid information and facts. But this time everything I researched led me in different directions and on a wild goose chase that left me more exhausted and frustrated. I wasn't doing myself any favours, but I also knew that self-education was the best way to track down what I needed, or thought I needed. I became an investigator, and an obsessive one at that. Day in and day out I researched, but every day led to the same conclusion. More confused, angry, exhausted, in pain, and even more devastated and depressed. Trying to wrap my head around what was going on with my health was the most difficult thing I have ever done.

My research began with Google searches around pain, exhaustion, and depression. My doctor had given me antidepressants, so naturally I looked up all I could on depression. Because I was in so much pain and entirely fatigued, these were also my initial search words. Did I tell anybody? Not a chance. Finding reliable and accurate resources about illness is like looking for a needle in a haystack. There are many many theories, books, doctors, authors, and scientific data on all of these subjects, which only left me more discouraged and led me in even more directions, from adrenal fatigue to burnout to chronic fatigue, major depression, and fibromyalgia. I was trying to prove to myself that there was a reason for my sickness outside of who I was. I wanted to find something or someone to blame for causing this in me. I continued to hear people say that they just push through when they are tired and get things done, and do what they have to do. But why couldn't I do the same anymore, when I had done it so many times in the past? I can't express enough how much this made me feel like a failure and was one of the main reasons that I withdrew from people. Sorting out why I was sick was going to be a bigger task than I thought and only compounded my loss of purpose and anxiety, because the more I learned, the more my gut told me I was really sick and that I would be off work longer. Narrowing down reliable sources to understand where I was at was a huge uphill battle and one that I really was in no shape to take on. But, hey, that's what we do, right? We need to make sense of why.

If only I just had had a list of go-to resources that could have made it easy for me to understand what was happening to my body. Did I say I lived on the internet? Oh yeah! Constantly reading – and I know driving my husband nuts by "educating" him. But really, I was trying to prove to him that I was sick and there was a good explanation for it.

It took me a long time to understand what led to me getting sick. Depression, fibromyalgia, and chronic fatigue are much more complex than even doctors know. Not everyone has the same symptoms at the same time or to the same degree. This is what is so puzzling to comprehend. There is no cookie cutter diagnosis or remedy, and this is why it takes so long to understand. I really want you to figure out what led to you getting sick and I hope to simplify the long process I had to take. I want you to begin to see this because it will help you to understand that it is not because of weakness that you are sick. I believe it is the opposite.

It is because you are so strong, so capable, and so driven that you continued to strive for success or perfection. I am also willing to bet that there were outside forces going on that you had no control over causing you even more stress. Loneliness, depression, fear, anxiety, pain, exhaustion, and despair slowly crept in without you seeing where you were headed and why you are now on sick leave trying to figure out how to get back to the job you love and to enjoy living.

First, stop frantically searching the internet and I will help you with reliable resources to narrow your search so that you can begin to understand what led to you getting sick.

I am not a doctor or health-care professional. This book will help you to do what you always do when you have a problem: search for answers, gather information, and make informed decisions based on evidence from reliable resources. Instead of you having to spend thousands of hours trying to make sense of all the confusion out there to only leave you more confused and at a loss, I can be your partner and resource to help simplify a process for you to sort out your symptoms and feelings and begin your own journey back to the career you love.

This chapter is only the tip of the iceberg of understanding. Don't give up and don't allow yourself to be overwhelmed. You've had enough of that and I only want to give you what you need at the moment. I want to give you enough to think about at the end of the day to start to understand what made you sick, but not so much that you don't want to think about it because it is too confusing. You're not alone. This book is for you, so that you can feel supported, understood, and have a pathway to empower you to take control again. I hope to take away the guilt, embarrassment, and feelings of failure that I know you have.

When you reflect on possible causes, do so only in a relaxed state and only long enough that you don't start to feel stressed or overwhelmed. Pretend you are outside of yourself looking down at yourself and seeing yourself for the first time as someone else might see you. What are you doing? What are you saying to yourself and others? What decisions do you need to make? How are you organizing all of the things that need to be done? What do you look like at work? What do you look like at home? Where do you feel the most exhausted? What gives you energy? What takes your energy? What makes you feel successful? What makes you feel like you're a failure? What gives you joy? What takes away joy? Where do you do your best thinking?

How do you stay focused? Who do you connect with on a professional level to collaborate? Do you take all tasks on yourself? Do you ever ask for help? Do you help others? Do you or are you able to say no? Can you say no at home but not at work? Can you say no at work but not at home? Do you see stress as something that motivates you and keeps you going? Do you see stress negatively affecting others but think that is not you? Do you know of anyone else who feels like you? Have you ever confided in someone about how you are feeling? Do you ever relax? Do you take vacations? Do you work 24/7? Do you bring work home? Do you do the work you bring home?

Asking yourself questions like these when you are on the outside looking in helps you to see yourself as others may see you. You may start to see yourself the way you look at others. It's difficult to take a look at ourselves and reflect, but I've learned from teaching that it is the best tool to self-discovery and growth.

Chapter 5:

Is It All in My Head?

Myth: *Fibromyalgia is not a real illness.*

Fact: *Fibromyalgia has been around for centuries but has evolved in name over time. The pain, fatigue, cognitive issues, and other symptoms are real and a diagnosis can be made. It's just not an easy process to get there.*

*I*f you're like I was, you're still trying to figure out all the crazy symptoms that seem to ebb and flow. They don't go away. They change and morph and you're left asking yourself, "What the heck is wrong with me?" Your brain starts to play tricks on you and fear creeps in. You begin to think "I must be really sick," especially after being off work for so long with no change. I was there too, and it was the most horrible feeling in the world. I began to hate going to bed every night, hoping and praying to feel different in the morning but waking up disappointed once again that nothing had changed. I read so much and even started to look at other diseases like MS, lupus, and rheumatoid arthritis, just to name a few. I was doing this and seeing my doctor as much as I could, but was at his mercy and hoping it was only depression because that would hopefully go away with medications. My doctor is wonderful and very supportive, especially when it comes to listening to patients. When a woman's gut instinct is speaking, he is very respectful and open to listening. This made it very easy to go to my regular appointments with him.

I found many of my symptoms described in many illnesses, but could not quite put my finger on which one fit. How much rest can one person need, really? All I did was lie on the couch, only to get up to put dinner on the table. Most days I would shower, but some days I just didn't have the energy to do it. I couldn't clean up after dinner because I was just that exhausted.

These are a list of the symptoms I was dealing with, and I am sure you are too. We may not have all the same ones – I have learned no two people will show exactly the same symptoms and it is why doctors have such a difficult time diagnosing fibromyalgia. Basically, they analyse your symptoms and rule out everything else, if they in fact get that far.

So the following are many of the symptoms people, mostly women, exhibit with fibromyalgia:

- Pain all over
- Over-sensitivity (not just emotionally)
- Stiffness
- Fatigue
- Poor sleep quality
- Cognitive problems (like a foggy brain)
- Headaches
- IBS (irritable bowel syndrome)
- Tender points

These are the most common, but you may also have:

- Dizziness
- Feeling too hot or too cold – you can't regulate your body temperature easily (Don't you love it when people tell you it's hot flashes and menopause?)
- Restless legs
- Tingling, numbness, or burning sensations in the hands and feet that feels like pins and needles
- Anxiety
- Depression (Who wouldn't be depressed, when you've felt so devastated for so long?)

Stay with me here. I don't want to overwhelm you, because if you are like I was, the more I researched and read the more overwhelmed and unhappy I became. Sorting out your symptoms seems simple enough at first. There are so many that you just start picking them off. It's like shooting fish in a barrel – no matter where you start you're bound to hit something. But you end up on a hamster wheel and going nowhere. When I was doing my teaching degree, we had an assignment where we had to come up with something to teach the rest of the class. I remember the class where a fellow student tried to teach us all how to juggle. There was a lot of laughing at first, but then focus and determination. Who wants to fail in front of all those fellow teacher candidates? Learning to figure out and attack your symptoms is somewhat like learning to juggle. You may already feel this way. I know it was for me. I would start with one symptom, add in another to try and manage, and then another, only to start dropping one of the "balls," feeling frustrated I couldn't get anywhere. Then I would give up and go back to lying on the couch, sleeping, watching TV, and feeling horrible about myself. Why couldn't I fix this? It looked easy: just manage one thing at a time. But sorting through these symptoms was not that easy. I needed to know what was wrong with me and why. I needed to know that I didn't cause this, although part of my brain was telling me I was a failure and just couldn't keep up – depression does that. That was not good for me or my symptoms. I also kept asking, "Why me?" Why did this have to happen when I was at a point in life that I had worked really hard to get to and now was finally in a position to love my job and really improve my financial position?

In the last chapter I mentioned a list of stressors and asked you questions about what you were doing in your life. While there are many thoughts, ideas, and theories on possible causes for fibromyalgia, as no one knows exactly what does cause it, I know mine was from chronic long-term stress with a traumatic incident that really put me over the edge.

I hope at this point you are starting to feel supported because someone actually gets what you're feeling and is willing to stay with you to get you on a better path.

When I was first off work, I had so many of the above symptoms that it was too overwhelming to even think about trying to help myself. My daily routine, as I hinted at earlier, was sleeping in, many days until eleven or so. If I could only get caught up on my sleep, I would be fine. But I had trouble going to sleep and it would be well past midnight some nights when I would finally sleep. I usually did not sleep through the night. A couple hours in, I would wake up, toss and turn. My best sleep usually came around four or five in the morning until late morning. I started to think that maybe just my circadian rhythm was screwed up. When I finally got up, my brain was so foggy that I couldn't think, let alone have a decent conversation or comprehend what was being said. Coffee was my best friend at that time of the day! It still is. Mornings are still somewhat tough, but I have made good improvements there, too. I've learned how to manage symptoms better, and I am confident you will as well.

So my symptoms included fatigue, brain fog, thinking issues, pain, and absolutely no energy or motivation for anything. It was coffee, couch, maybe some lunch, couch and nap, shower around four sometimes, and start dinner so that I gave the impression I was okay and could manage the house. This was way too much pressure on myself, which I now see, but I was doing myself no favours trying to look like I could do it all. I still believed that all I needed was rest and maybe the antidepressants would eventually make me feel something.

My brain fog and thinking issues were so bad that I could not even read for pleasure anymore. I could not retain a paragraph, let alone a page of text. But boy could I research online. I was obsessed with finding out what was wrong with me, reading and searching but not sharing this with anyone. I know I gave my husband lots of information on a daily basis. I was trying to prove to him that I was sick and that this was a real illness. I hadn't been diagnosed with fibromyalgia yet, so I was talking to him about anything and everything I read about that matched what I was feeling. I came across many things and considered many illnesses. When I came across adrenal fatigue, I finally felt I hit on something. There were many similarities, but I had never heard of this. It just sounded better than saying I was burnt out or that I had depression. Boy, was I adding to the stigma of each of these. I'm sure you've considered all sorts of illnesses, only to become more frustrated with not having a definitive answer with a definitive cure.

I'm sure my doctor got frustrated with me coming up with new labels. But I was desperate for answers so I could get to some solutions. I mentioned adrenal fatigue. He listened but never really gave me a diagnosis or label. He kept telling me I needed rest and to keep up with the antidepressants. I know we tried a few different ones as well.

I continued on this path for three years. I tried lots of things, from walking more to yoga classes to trying to meditate. While I loved the yoga classes, they were also exhausting. I tried to walk with friends, but I was just too tired to keep at this. It was much easier to stay inside and lay on the couch trying to read about all these illnesses. I really thought I was starting to hone in on something, but what was it?

I began to think that I was going to have to live like this the rest of my life, and that was a very discouraging and depressing thought. I was already depressed enough and felt like I was climbing out of an endless hole that kept piling in on me.

I am much better than I was then, but still work at managing my symptoms so that I can live life happily and work at a job I love. I could have gotten to this point much sooner had I known someone or had my doctor known what was wrong with me and how exactly I could begin to climb back to be me again. So where did I begin and what did I have to tackle first? For about three years I was trying to get caught up on my rest so I didn't feel tired all the time. I tried yoga classes, meditation classes, spending time sitting outdoors in nice weather, seeing my doctor on a regular basis, massage, acupuncture, a naturopathic doctor, and researching, researching, researching. I was spinning my wheels on this up and down journey and had no road map in front of me to guide me.

By now you're maybe looking at the above-mentioned symptoms saying yes to some or many and beginning to think that fibromyalgia is what you're dealing with. I asked my doctor for referrals to rheumatologists because that is what I read about online that many people went to. He continued to tell me that I didn't need to see one because I was not a candidate to be referred. This was indeed frustrating because I trusted my doctor, so I believed he knew what was best for me. But I only continued to be in pain, exhausted, devastated, and depressed. I really was trying anything that I thought might help, but was doing so without the support I actually needed.

Your symptoms are real. I want you to know that! They are not in your head as you may have already been told. They are real. In order to start your journey to something better you need to be open to learning about fibromyalgia, depression, and anxiety but keeping it simple and not overwhelming yourself. Fibromyalgia is a complicated illness that even the medical and alternative communities still find complex. You can feel better!

Chapter 6:

Why Do I Feel So Alone?

Myth: *You look good so you must be feeling better.*

Fact: *Fibromyalgia symptoms are confusing and invisible. They are not the same for everyone.*

Probably the worst feelings I had – not the worst symptom, but the worst feelings – were the loss of purpose and identity along with feeling so alone. I truly believe that, had my employer understood the signs that were pointing to me going downhill, that I would not have ended up as sick as I was. Maybe a lot of it could have been prevented. I will never know that for certain, but it is a gut feeling. By now you have a good idea of what led to you getting sick, just how confusing and complex fibromyalgia is, and all that can come with it. Just think: if it's confusing and complex to you, then expecting others to get it or understand is a stretch. Think about all the research you've been doing, all the sites you've been surfing and possibly the books you've been buying. You're still frustrated, and you've become an expert at researching fibromyalgia!

Right now, I want you to do yourself a huge favour. Stop trying to justify, explain, or prove your illness! Let me hold that for you for now.

Feeling alone did not hit really hard at first. I think it was because I thought I would return to work after a good rest and some meds in a few months' time. Boy, was I wrong. I'm sure you get that and it's likely one of the reasons you are reading this. You're at your wits' end and willing to do anything to take this bull by the horns and be you again.

Life is full of joys, triumphs, successes, and heartbreaks that are painful to bear. We all have them. What makes it hard is when someone else's pain, hurt, injury, or illness is compared to yours to minimize what you're going through, especially with illnesses that have stigmas attached to them, that the medical community has not fully embraced or acknowledged, and that are invisible. This was part of why I started to feel so alone.

I tried to stay in touch with coworkers, but when it ended up being me reaching out to them, I just stopped trying. It was exhausting for me anyway and I just couldn't keep doing it. I was doing my best to still be their friend for whatever they were going through, but when it felt like it was just me reaching out to them then I started to wonder what was wrong with me. I was negative about me and my situation. I didn't know that who I had become was actually a combination of symptoms of other illnesses that can accompany fibromyalgia or crop up before a diagnosis of fibromyalgia is given.

I felt so alone that I was beginning to not leave the house as much. I preferred to take a small walk alone or with my husband. Any of the yoga or other classes I attended were in a different city because I didn't want to run into anyone I knew. I felt alone because I needed my friends and family to still care and reach out to help me. I wanted them to understand and not look at me with pity. I hated that when I saw it. I did not have the ability to be there for anyone else anymore.

The last thing you need now is advice. Advice on pain, advice on sleep, advice on exercise, advice on food, because what this ends up doing is overwhelming you with more stuff to consider. You've already read enough about your symptoms and what you might think they are. After all, you know your own body better than anyone and your gut will guide you as well.

I spent a lot of time feeling I had to prove my illness because "I didn't look sick." Oh, but yes I did. I didn't let people see me looking bad. Who does that?! What they should have noticed is that they were not seeing me as much. They didn't realize when they did see me that I looked good because it took me hours to get ready and get my energy up to socialize and see people.

The hero attitude that society has driven into us over the last few decades is killing us. The thinking now that if you're constantly busy, tired, and have no time you must be a very successful person. You often wonder how these people do it. Not too long ago, it was ideal for the woman to be at home raising children while her spouse worked. When women started to enter the workforce, that was stigmatized as you were supposed to be home. We've come a long way since then. I think the opposite may be true now, but many women have only dumped more on their shoulders trying to do it all instead of balancing life so that they are healthy and happy. The thinking that if you can't do it all, then there must be something wrong with you and you're a failure is wrong. This is what is making us sick and feel alone, because in reality, that's *not* reality. Add on an illness that is confusing and invisible, and you really are alone.

So right now, stop trying to prove to anybody what you have. Stop trying to justify your reasons for having to take sick leave. By the way, these feelings only intensify when you need to go on long-term disability. (If you're at that point and need to apply now, I can help you with this, too.) I didn't realize how much this is looked down upon until I had to do it. Yes, that's how long I ended up off work. When I had to apply for long-term disability because my short-term sick leave was running out, I was so upset because once again I was a failure, or so I thought. This meant that I was going to be off of work for up to two years and have a further reduced income. Talk about stress – and just when I didn't need any more! If you have to take sick leave, insurance companies are not as supportive as you might think or have planned for. God forbid you get something that they think doesn't exist or think that if you just walk more you will be fine.

Sick leave and disability insurance are there to support people. When you know someone who is off, do everything you can to reach out to them and just be there. Listen to them and just be there. What people need the most is compassion, understanding, and empathy. I had one person who never gave up on me. She knows who she is, and she also knows that whatever she has to deal with in life, I will also listen – I owe her that. She doesn't realize that each time she called, emailed, or texted she was giving me a lifeline that kept me afloat just when I thought I was going to sink. I am forever grateful to her.

Loneliness with this illness comes from our own negative thinking. That's due in part to the depression/anxiety piece, and in part to what society has driven us to believe. It comes from not being able to reach out to others anymore. It comes from others not understanding or trying to learn all they can to understand. It comes from you ending up not having the energy or desire to get out there anymore.

"But you don't look sick?" "You look good, you must be feeling better." Oh, do I detest hearing these. I did end up telling people, "I have good days and bad days." I didn't quite know what to say because I was still not being honest with myself about depression and fibromyalgia. When others have their own opinions about why you're off sick it can be really hard to bite your tongue to not scream at them. I still struggle with people's questions and push myself to get out and socialize, but it is easier now. You will get there too.

I think the biggest "alone" feeling was trying to be the mom my kids had always known. That was really hard. I could only imagine what they thought. I know they were worried, but they never ever let it show. To this day I still feel guilty I somehow let them down because I couldn't be that mom anymore.

Saying "*No!*" can also be really tough, especially when you loved visiting with others and hosting family at home. I just couldn't do what I used to do, and yes, that made me feel alone. Thank goodness my mom and aunt could see how sick I was. We started sharing special holidays so it was not as much work for any of us. That meant store-bought dessert and simpler dishes, but in the end it only mattered that we were still together. This was another hard thing for me to relinquish. I loved making desserts and cooking for family, especially the turkey dinners. I felt guilty too, and I know you are feeling that right now. Again, stop please and step back. Evaluate what really matters so you don't feel alone.

My career definitely defined who I was. It took me years to fulfil that dream and landing my dream job was like winning the lottery and I had felt so blessed to have been hired. Some say lucky. Nope! I worked hard, really hard, to prove that I was the best candidate.

Having my career define who I was as a person is not something I recommend to anyone. I did not realize I even felt this way until I was not teaching. I was devastated and was grieving the loss of me. That was the most alone I felt on this journey. I began to consider other careers. My new research obsession was other careers/jobs. I had applications out all over the place! I took two interviews to really great positions, only to be told they hired internally.

If you're doing this like I did, I don't recommend staying on that path. It didn't help me to feel better about myself. It only made me feel worse and more and more alone. As I look back, I was trying to prove that I was still successful. I felt I needed to prove my worth.

I really want you to know that you are not alone. Fibromyalgia, depression, anxiety, and any invisible illness are extremely confusing to understand and even more complex to treat. You know so much more than you realize, and you are capable of so much more as well. You just need an easier road map to get to where you want to be than the one I used. You are not alone in your confusion and understanding of what made you sick. It just feels like that, but you can feel better. I've created this plan of attack to help you shorten the time you need to feel better in order to get back to the job you love or the career you do not want to give up. I did it and so can you.

Chapter 7:

How Do I Get Stuff Done and Focus on Being Well?

Myth: *Having a good day means*
I can get more stuff done.

Fact: *Trying to get more stuff done on a good day*
usually leads to a setback and symptoms flare.

*L*et's start getting you feeling some success. All it takes is some little adjustments, and you will be surprised just how good that makes you start to feel. I felt so out of control in my life that I was spinning and didn't know which way to turn. I will talk about doctors, etc. in the next chapter, but for now I want you to have some simple things to do so that you can feel in control and start to feel some relief.

I hope by now you realize how much I have said rest. Rest, rest, rest! This is what you really need to make sure you get. I know you're saying, "But I have all these other things to do!" Yup, and they will still be there after you rest. Maybe you do already rest but are confused when, a couple days later, you feel like you're back to square one, exhausted again. That's because you are. You're overdoing it on those days because you feel good and think you need to play catch-up to what you couldn't do. I look at my energy like a cell phone battery. My battery is no longer brand new and it drains really quickly and doesn't stay charged as long. I still work at this, but I am so much better at it than before and have improved as a result.

All the day-to-day stuff was way too overwhelming for me, so I ended up back on the couch. But when you have a plan of attack on the day-to-day stuff, it can make a whole lot of difference.

I found this very hard because it meant I had to admit to myself that I could not do what I used to do. I still had those voices in my head saying, "You can do this," and the voices out there saying "Just push through, we all get tired" or whatever variation you hear.

Did I say rest yet? Number one priority is to rest. As soon as you start to feel tired, you need to rest. Even if it means resting all day, listen to your body for cues telling you it needs a break and rest.

Asking for Help

Okay, next I want you to *ask for help*! I know, people like you and I tend to not want to or ever ask for help because we have always just finished what we needed to do. Now is not one of those times. It is essential to ask for help. Who do you ask first and what do you ask for? This may take some reflection on your part, but if you only pick one thing that's absolutely fine. It means you are doing something and moving forward toward improvement. The best thing I did for myself was to hire cleaning ladies. Actually, I've had cleaning ladies for most of my life because I have always worked full time. Even when I had to scrimp and save to have them, it was the best investment for me and my family. It takes the pressure off of who is going to do all the cleaning, major stuff anyway. You might have to not expect things to be perfect. I could never quite get my house perfect, but I know some people who do and for the life of me, I don't have a clue how they do it. Laundry can be easily taken care of by each family member doing their own. This is a great skill for children to learn, especially teenagers. It just might mean they don't bring home dirty laundry on weekends when they go to university.

It is really important to be open and honest with your spouse and children about what you are going through. I know my family worried *so* much. I wish I had known how to talk to them so they could understand, but it was tough enough for me to get what was going on. Start by talking about one symptom and then go from there. Don't talk for too long, as your brain is likely having a tough time keeping track at this point. But having your husband understand what you're going through will make it so much easier for you to get the help and support you need. If you're like me, you love to make your house a home for your family. Having to give up some of that was hard, but it was essential. I really didn't have a choice. So sitting down and talking about how family members can help will not only take a weight off of your shoulders but will help to give you the necessary time to get in the rest you need.

Keeping Up with Others – Don't Do It!

My husband has so much energy and this was a challenge for me. I had that kind of energy until I got sick. I continued to try and keep up and didn't tell him exactly how it affected me. That was the wrong thing to do. It broke my heart not to be able to keep up anymore. I am better with that now, but it took some time to get there. Once he understood and saw for himself what I was going through, then he was even able to help me not overdo it. When you start to think about how you burn energy, you will be surprised when you realize how much is burned just thinking about what you can't do. I found if I had a lot of thinking tasks, I was too tired to add in physical tasks and vice versa. So let it go and understand it's okay if he has energy to burn. Give him more tasks around the house to keep him busy. Staying one step ahead, thinking about projects for him to complete can be tiring as well. Have a list of things that need to be accomplished that he hasn't had time to get to.

Paying Bills and Handling Finances

I am the financial planner of the household. I would gladly give it up, but my husband is more than happy to let me do it. We do work together on goals and things to spend money on, but for the majority of the finances I take care of them. To simplify this, I paid bills on the days we got paid and had a budget for everything else. That was necessary anyway, because my income had significantly dropped. Setting this up is essential and also takes the worry out of what gets paid when and keeping track of it. Setting up automatic withdrawals for regular bills works really well too, as it is one less thing to have to think about and do. Make sure they are scheduled around the day before they are due so you avoid late fees/penalties as well. I also only did this on payday and then progressed to one day a week. This saves you more time – and guess what you're going to do with that time? You guessed it, rest!

Climbing Stairs

Stairs were difficult for me. I can remember it taking time to climb them. This may sound strange, but when I realized how much energy I burned up by taking the stairs too much, I started to plan to reduce the number of times I had to do so in a day. If you have stairs in your home or a second floor you may have realized this already. Today I can actually use our stairs multiple times in the day and I sometimes have the energy to *run* up them. I remember the first time I could do this. I actually did it without thinking and then I thought, "Wow, I haven't been able to do that for so long. I must be improving." This should happen for you as well. But it takes time by managing your energy and daily step count. The thing to remember is to be conscious of the reason you're having to use the stairs and try your very best to minimize this throughout the day.

Daily Routines

Daily routines are somewhat more complicated because it is difficult to have a routine when you don't know how you're going to feel on any given day. In the beginning I slept and rested a lot. I would say that for a good three years, this was my life. I know I could have shortened that time had I not had to figure all of this out by trial and error and, eventually, with a coach, but I will talk more about that in the next chapter. Flexibility is essential if you want to be able to build back routines and structure into your daily life. You may have difficulty with this, especially if you still have children at home. But that's when you empower them to take on more responsibility. Give them small jobs at first and little things to help out with, depending on their age of course. When they start to see how it helps you, they will embrace it more.

Grocery Shopping and Shopping in General

I am not a shopper, so shopping was easy to not do. But we still needed to eat, so grocery shopping was a necessity. I felt like I should be able to do it, considering I wasn't working, but again, that was not what I should have been thinking. For me, grocery shopping was extremely difficult during this time. I still have issues with it but have come to terms with my abilities now and developed some good strategies. None of us starved and we still ate well. But I could not cook the way I used to. I needed to simplify. I remember going to the grocery store. I wouldn't get far before I would have to turn around and go home. It was much too overwhelming for me and overstimulating. I can't tell you how many times I did that. So, I asked for help. My husband started to go with me. But even with his help it was too overwhelming and exhausting to do a full grocery shop. We started small and shopped for one meal, and other times he would stop in on his way home to pick up a few things.

I began to see a naturopath (more on that in the next chapter), and because I eliminated gluten, dairy, eggs, and fruit, meal prep became easier. Every day I was essentially eating meat and vegetables and having two protein shakes that my doctor prescribed. This was a life saver. It meant I only had to think about one meal. I still felt I had to get dinner together, and it was the only accomplishment I was able to do. It felt wonderful having dinner ready for my husband when he got home. He was so supportive on so many things that I could at least do this. He was also willing to eat what I did, unless he decided to add to the meal. A couple times a week he picked up supplies to cook, and we went out as well to take some pressure off. Surprisingly, this gave me more time to rest. I didn't have a choice, because my body was dictating that. There was no pushing through. My husband also cleaned up after supper, and this, again, was very helpful. I was usually too tired anyway and had to lie down.

Meal Planning

Planning meals was also difficult, and I was not able to plan more than two days out. Sometimes I could only manage to plan one dinner. So that's what I did. When I was able to go to the grocery store, I started with just the vegetable and meat sections. That was easy to choose for a couple of dinners. Then I progressed to the outside aisles of the store when necessary. That's where all the food that is necessary for healthy meals is anyway, but the real reason was that it was too overwhelming to go through all the other aisles. It still is at times, but I am able to do it better now. Surprisingly, this routine saved us money on groceries. I didn't buy at whim going throughout the store. I got what I needed and got out because I was usually very tired by then and needed to get home to rest. I usually timed going right after lunchtime. I did this so that I could get back and have a rest before I needed to start prepping dinner. At that time, I was not able to do more than one errand at a time on any given day. Running errands was really taxing on my body and brain. As I said, I could not do more than one and I had to have a day in-between to stay home and rest. I only learned this through trial and error, but it took a long time to see what worked and what the pattern was for draining my energy.

Social Activities

Attending events and functions was also difficult, because it was so exhausting just to get ready to go anywhere that by the time we left, I was already tired and needing rest.

We stayed home a lot and made lots of excuses for why we couldn't do things. There were times when I did overdo it and paid dearly the next day. You will likely have to pick and choose and plan which things you go to and have the strength to say no. It's for the best when trying to improve your symptoms. It also meant having company was almost out of the question. Visiting with anyone anywhere took a lot out of me. I would go home and crash after. One strategy I did use was to arrive just before things started and, when possible, leave early. It was not ideal, but it was necessary. Also, when visiting, make the visits shorter so that you accomplish two things: seeing people and not draining your energy as badly.

Showering, Getting Dressed, and Doing Makeup:

I mentioned what I did about this in an earlier chapter. There were many times that I had to rest after a shower and would often skip a day in-between because it tired me out. There were times I would lie down after having a shower, before being able to get dressed and do my hair and makeup. Often I would have to rest again after getting dressed and doing my hair and makeup. When I started listening to when my body needed to rest, I began discovering patterns and triggers to the pain and fatigue.

Cognitive Issues

My cognitive issues were quite noticeable, to me anyway. I am sure others noticed changes, but to hide them I withdrew and/or was quieter when out with people, because

I really was limited on having good conversations. It was exhausting for me and I felt stupid for not being able to carry on conversations the way I used to or felt I should. I was limited to talking about my kids, the weather, and simple things. I was on edge that questions about my health would surface and I wouldn't know what to say, but it was also exhausting having conversations, and I was reluctant to share what was actually going on. I felt like I had to defend myself. This alone stopped me from going places. I know I stumbled over various excuses instead of just saying what I had, considering I did not have a clear diagnosis on anything other than that I was taking antidepressants, I was exhausted and in pain, and having cognitive issues. I had not yet been diagnosed with fibromyalgia. I didn't want to share and felt it made me look weak and that I was making excuses for being off work. I've come a long way since then and become more accepting of the diagnoses I have received. I have to ask though, why are we so cruel to each other depending on what illness you have?

Reading

Another difficulty was reading. I guess it was the brain fog and cognitive issues. I love to read and research, however the only reading I did was online, obsessively searching for answers. I was unable to read for pleasure. I tried so much at bedtime to do this, as I hoped it would help me get to sleep. But I only got more frustrated. I was not able to retain what I was reading and would have to reread paragraphs and pages. I eventually gave up. TV and web searching were it.

Friends

I talked about feeling alone in the last chapter, and this just became more and more of a problem as I pulled away or people drifted away. I had one friend who never gave up on me. When I was still working, she saw what was happening to me and was really concerned. In fact, we had not been close at work but knew each other well enough. When she reached out to me, she could have as easily stopped just as much as get in touch again. But she didn't. Since that first phone call she has been a shoulder to cry on, a loyal friend, someone who listened and really understood how bad I was, and someone to laugh with. To this day she is still that same person. She never gave up on me and continued to reach out when I was unable to be the one doing the reaching, even when she was going through difficult times. I will forever be there for her and she knows that. I'm not sure I will ever be able to repay her, but I know that whenever she needs me she knows she can call and I'm glad to say she has. No matter what, she knows that I am always and will always be there for her. All it takes is one friend through times like these. You need it too. And do not be afraid to reach out to someone. You might be surprised who ends up being that person for you. I know I was and because of it have been blessed with one of the best friendships of my life.

Getting a handle on the day-to-day stuff is essential to starting your journey to enjoy life and have a goal of getting back to work. The biggest thing to remember is that it takes baby steps. Very, very small baby steps. That takes discipline to do, but you must.

These suggestions are what helped me to start taking back some of that control that I so missed.

Chapter 8:

Treatments – Traditional, Alternative, or Both?

Myth: Fibromyalgia is curable.

Fact: There is no magic pill for fibromyalgia and no cure at this point. It takes time and a balanced approach of many treatment options to find what works best for you.

*T*rying to navigate the medical and alternative medicine worlds is confusing at best. There is so much conflicting information in books, between doctors, and as we all know, on the internet. We have so much information at our fingertips now that it can be scary to read up on things. On top of this are the people in our lives who also have "knowledge" and opinions about you being sick. When you're living with a foggy brain, exhausted, and in pain, the last thing you need is someone telling you what to do or trying to make sense of the labyrinth of information you continue to research and gather. I bet you're no further ahead than you were a year ago. My hope is that the practical approach I'm sharing in this book helps you to narrow your search down and provides you with information that you can feel confident in turning to and use to begin to unravel your own issues so you can move toward returning to the life you love.

This chapter focuses on traditional and alternative approaches to reduce your symptoms and get you on a path to wellness and joy.

I will refer to many health-care professionals in this chapter, but by no means is it an exhaustive list. These are the ones that I consulted or sought out before I finally was able to make sense of where I needed to start. I really hope that by doing this I can shorten the time you are off work and back to a life you love.

Your family doctor is the place to start, as you would with any medical symptoms. The first step you've taken is to take sick leave so you can first and foremost get some rest. Please don't disregard the suggestion of antidepressants, but only take them under your doctor's care. This is common with the symptoms that took you to the doctor in the first place. I will discuss more on this in a bit, but for now do not rule out what your doctor is trying to do.

What Came First: Depression or Fibromyalgia?

Depression alone is a horrible illness to manage and comes with stigma. Taking medication is a must, but people in general will make comments like "Oh, I don't believe in taking medication," or "That's not for me." This boggles my mind because they are not doctors nor do I think they have a solid understanding of what depression is and how it must be treated and managed. Fibromyalgia has enough horrible symptoms that depression definitely is part of it. Being depressed and having depression are also different. Being depressed can come and go and it's become a common term to use when just feeling down or even sad. But major depression is much worse. The low mood never leaves and robs you of the ability to feel joy. Due to the nature of symptoms from fibromyalgia, it's no wonder depression often accompanies fibromyalgia. But sometimes it's hard to figure out which came first. Fibromyalgia can lead to depression while depression does not necessarily lead to fibromyalgia.

Understanding fibromyalgia and depression/anxiety and finding treatments begins with shooting darts at the dartboard and then moving on from there. I really did think my career was over. I was sick to my stomach over this. I actually didn't think I'd ever work again, let alone teach. These thoughts only made my mood decline. I know this is a symptom of the depression, but it is something I am conscious of. Many of the things that help manage fibromyalgia symptoms also help depression symptoms. Depression and fibromyalgia are often diagnosed together and this is why many of these strategies help both.

Psychiatry

I did a lot of self-reflecting to determine what my very worst symptom was and thought I would try and focus on that first. My thinking was that if I could do something about that, then maybe I could begin to work on other symptoms one at a time to get myself to a place where I could make sound decisions about my career. I felt my worst symptom was depression and, as it turned out, that was the case. This step was the first step back for me. Up until this point I was chasing symptoms like I was playing whack-a-mole and I'd just get one looking like it might be managed and then another would flare up worse. I was lucky that my psychiatrist was so caring and involved in my path back to wellness. One of the first things she sent me to do was the sleep study I mentioned before. Difficulty sleeping is one of the fibro symptoms that keep you in a state of endless pain and fatigue. You need sleep to help with pain, but pain keeps you awake. While I did not look like a candidate for sleep apnea, we were surprised to learn that I was having apneas and would need to try a CPAP machine. I wasn't getting the type of sleep necessary to feel refreshed. This is one area in which I am continuing to work on with doctors.

I was prescribed something to help me get to sleep by my psychiatrist and then she made major changes to the medications I was taking for depression, anxiety, and pain. I was reluctant because you hear so many people say "I won't take meds. I don't want to get hooked or rely on them." I used to think that. I had many medication trials and changes. During the course of these medication tweaks and changes, my doctor asked me to take part in psychodynamic therapy. I didn't even know what that was. She explained it was an in-depth form of talk therapy used to treat depression and that it works well for those who have lost meaning in their lives. This made sense to me and I was willing to try anything. I began with weekly appointments and would be in the program for about a year.

It took months for my psychiatrist to get the perfect mix of prescriptions for me to feel something different. I can remember the day when I thought something was different. I had been seeing the doctor for almost a year at this point and was still desperately hoping for something to work. We were on vacation visiting friends and I said to my husband, "I feel something different with this last medication change. I'm not sure what it is, but it's different." I was afraid to jinx myself, but I was certain something was happening. This was July, 2017, and on my next follow-up in August I was actually feeling that maybe I could consider going back to work. I couldn't believe I was thinking this, because I had not had any inkling at all whatsoever for any purpose in my life. This was a step in the right direction.

Chiropractor

In the fall of 2016, I noticed an ad in the paper one day for a chiropractor who had helped someone with fibromyalgia. I was interested in getting more information, so I set up an appointment. Just like I was when I finally got to the psychiatrist, I was in a very bad place when I had my first appointment with the chiropractor. I was in tears in his office just looking for something to give me hope. His approach is to educate his patients before even starting treatment and I really liked this because it helped me to really understand how chiropractic work could be very beneficial for me. He set up a treatment plan for me where I had to see him three days a week at first, then we tapered off to once a week. It took time, but I gradually started to notice that there were improvements to my body and that chiropractic adjustments helped to reduce my all over pain, particularly in certain areas where I had higher pain levels. I have continued my weekly appointments and I continue to see how I am still improving with his help.

I firmly believe chiropractic work is essential to managing fibromyalgia, but you need to find the right chiropractor for you. It takes time to see results and you must be willing to be patient to feel this. When you are finally in a good place, you will then bounce back much faster from flare-ups than you did prior to having treatments.

Naturopathic Doctor

This is another health care professional that I believe has been instrumental in my symptom management. I found one who had a traditional medical background who then went on to study naturopathic medicine. This seems to be a great combination to getting sound advice. My doctor was very familiar with adrenal fatigue, fibromyalgia, depression, and anxiety. Like chiropractic work, this modality takes time but is well worth being patient to see and feel results.

Chapter 9:

Am I Really Starting to Feel Better?

Myth: Fibromyalgia symptoms
cannot be improved.

Fact: You can improve symptoms
when you work with someone
who's been there.

I promise you will eventually start to make improvements,
but trying to do it all at once doesn't work.
Baby steps are the key to success with this illness.

Massage

*A*hhhhhh, massage! Who doesn't love massage? If you haven't tried it, do it. This is a treatment that must be included in order to manage symptoms. Do you remember the first pedicure you had and what that felt like? Well, this feeling is even better than that. If you're nervous and don't know where to find someone, ask around. Chances are many people you know see a massage therapist on a regular basis. Many health benefits plans cover you for massage therapy by a registered massage therapist. Check that out for sure. Some massage therapists will even let you bring in your partner so they can teach them some techniques to get you through between appointments. I know this has worked for me. At first massage will be exhausting and can continue to be so. But the benefits are worth it. Finding the right therapist requires trial and error to find one who understands fibromyalgia and what helps and what doesn't.

This is a must for me now. I was advised to find a massage therapist who was trained in the John Barnes method. This only took a quick Google search and I found only one trained therapist in my area. This method is done without the use of oil and focuses on stretching out the fascia. This is the thin layer of connective tissue in-between your skin and muscles. Some research has shown that this is where some of the pain in fibromyalgia is stemming from. Since learning this, I have been able to pinpoint this pain and know when I need to see my massage therapist. When I had to find a therapist closer to my work, I had my massage therapist refer me to someone she knew could still help me. My new massage therapist uses a cupping technique by dragging the cups up and down the muscles. This can be done with different tensions so it doesn't flare the pain. It took a couple of tries to find the correct tension, but once that was established, I began to look forward to my treatments. I have a regular monthly routine of meeting with my massage therapist and this works really well to keep my symptoms managed.

Energy

I also needed to get my energy (or lack thereof) under control, and one of the tips I learned from my fibromyalgia advising course was to monitor my step count. This was a game changer and so simple. Most phones have a step counter, so I began to track my steps. I also kept track of what I did and how I felt daily. This helped me to see patterns emerge and realize just how much rest was essential for me now. I couldn't believe how few steps I was able to take before exhaustion crept in. At first I was only doing about a thousand steps a day. That's not a typo, you read it right. One thousand steps was all I was able to do, and some days I couldn't do that much. Remember the comparison I made between my energy and a cell phone battery? This exercise of counting my steps is how I realized this was true. Many days, just going up and down a flight of stairs in our home too many times would take too much of my energy. Exercise for those of us with fibromyalgia is somewhat of a double-edged sword. Exercise can help, but too much can hurt. For me, too many steps in a day could cause a setback and I would have worse symptoms for a day or so and sometimes longer. This explained why I was so exhausted on my trip to China. I was defeating my own purpose of trying to walk ten thousand steps or more, only to figure out that was actually hurting me more. Managing steps was one of the best things I did for myself. While it was frustrating to only be able to accomplish about one thousand, it also answered why I was drained of energy all the time. This took time to improve and by the time I started back to work in February, 2018, I was only able to do about twelve hundred or so steps a day without exhausting myself. But at least I could see some small improvements. I made sure I did not have any appointments after school on back-to-back days so that I could average out my steps. Gradually this began to improve. I remember one evening that winter I thought we could try skiing again. After only an hour on the slopes, I was exhausted. I looked at my step count and it was around 1,500 and I knew I couldn't continue. My husband was so patient, loving, and kind and supported my recovery one hundred percent. I could not have accomplished all that I have without his support.

This was a start and gave me the chance to set small achievable goals and to analyse what and how much worked well and what didn't. I am now able to manage about 6,000 to 6,500 steps depending on the day, and when I go over, I can feel the same exhaustion. There are some days where only 3,500 steps are doable. When this happens, I know I have to get some rest. Nothing else matters. The rest is the most important thing I can do when I overdo it.

Music

This can be both positive and negative for you. When I'm feeling down, listening to music I love can be really helpful, especially for my mood. Choose music that you love that is upbeat and motivational. When it makes you feel like you want to get up and dance, then you're on the right track with music. It wasn't until I had the depression symptoms managed that I was able to use music for everything else. This may take some trial and error on your part. Try to pay attention to how music you listen to makes you feel. You'll be surprised at the effect if you've not done this before.

Restless Legs

I realized that while sleeping my legs were restless enough to wake me or keep me from getting a good sleep. This, too, is common in fibromyalgia patients. I learned that magnesium oil can help. I ordered mine online from a good reputable company. To use it, you mix it with water as described on the label. In a spray bottle (a dollar store purchase), the solution looks just like water and sprays just like water. When I know or think my legs might bother me, I just spray a little on and rub it in. It works! For me, anyway. I also recently suggested it to my father who was having leg cramps at night. He found relief as well. This is a simple, drug-free way to get some relief from restless legs at night.

Exercise

I am still working on this one, but managing fibromyalgia symptoms along with depression is a balancing act and means putting your self-care first. It's the only way to make the climb back to having the life you want and getting back to the career you love. I mentioned at the beginning of the chapter that managing my steps was necessary to figure out where and how much my energy would burn out. The key to this is not to go past the threshold you've established when you have gone too far, only to exhaust yourself and set yourself back a few days. It will happen, but don't give up. These setbacks eventually become farther apart and fewer as long as you listen and pay attention to your body. A year ago, I could only ski for one hour and only went once. But this past New Year's, we went away for a few days to a ski resort. I was stunned that I was able to ski again. I made sure I took breaks and didn't ski quite as hard as I used to. But this was a huge improvement in just one year. I still struggle with the fatigue. It's not as bad, but it still hinders my motivation to exercise. This is something that I will continue to work on but not stress over. I know it will come because the past year has been so enlightening on how to manage and move forward.

Yoga

If you have not tried yoga, I highly recommend it. It is great exercise and it really helps with pain relief and improves your mindset. Sticking to it seems to be the hardest part, but you may find that is easy for you. So far, yoga has been the best all-around form of relief for all of my symptoms. You may find this, too. Just don't rely on it solely. As I have mentioned, it takes multiple approaches to improve and stay well.

Meditation

Meditation alleviates stress and helps you to focus on the present. I learned this from going to yoga classes that have a focus on meditation and then taking a meditation course. I recommend trying it, but suggest embracing the meditation part of the yoga classes before taking on a meditation course. The biggest thing is not to take on too much all at once. I was trying to do that, and it didn't work. I was only more stressed that things were not working – and back on the hamster wheel. Only when I stepped back, took on the worst symptom, and had patience to move forward that I eventually learned how to find relief and make some improvements in my life.

Heat

Heat feels wonderful for my muscles and body pain. I am fortunate to have a hot tub, and this really helps to alleviate the pain, even for a short period of time. If you don't have a hot tub, a hot bath with Epsom salts is great, too. I often have a hotter shower if I don't have time to get in the hot tub and that will even give me some relief. Dry summertime heat feels awesome, too. I sunburn very easily so I am careful of how long I sit in direct sun, but just being outside in the heat does help me a great deal. When it gets really humid, I do tend to have increased pain though, and the regular massage appointment helps. Massage helps to keep symptoms in a good place, but only with regularly scheduled appointments.

Rest

This is still very, very important for me. I tend to push myself, but I have learned that I can't do that. I still do it from time to time and sometimes make the conscious choice to do something even if I know I will be in pain and exhausted for a day or two after. Those setbacks are just that, small setbacks. Once you take charge and focus your attention getting back to symptom management as soon as possible after, small setbacks can be worth it. Things that are really important to you like family dinners and getting together with friends, as well as staying up too late, and eating the wrong foods are just some things you may choose to overextend on, knowing you will have to take extra self-care for a few days to get back on track. The times that I overdo it now are fewer and farther between, because I choose those times and pay attention more to symptom management. When I was first starting to make progress moving forward, overdoing it was one of the easiest things to set me back because I was still trying to do all the things I used to. I would get so tired it felt like I was hitting a wall and I had to lie down and rest or sleep right away. Over the past year I have been able to increase my ability to do things for longer periods of time, but I really have to make sure that I attend to self-care and rest. This is especially true on weekends after working all week. Weekends can be busy, and when they are, it does force me to step back and recharge again.

Mornings

These were and still are the worst for me, and I am betting you're having difficulty with mornings too. Coffee was and still is my best friend. It takes me a couple of hours to get going, as I need that time to get my brain working like I need it to. I still don't wake up feeling refreshed, but am waiting for another sleep study to work on this. I don't sleep until ten or eleven anymore, and I don't require afternoon naps, although sometimes I am so tired after work I will have a rest before starting dinner. This used to be daily when I first started back to work; now it is less often. My brain is foggiest in the morning, and sometimes that fog hangs on throughout the day. It used to be all day and every day, but time and learning that my self-care affects this has helped me to focus on that so that I can be at my best (whatever that is for the day). I go to bed at ten p.m. and now set my alarm for eight thirty a.m. Sometimes I wake up earlier, but it is best if I sleep at least until then. This has been a big improvement. I continue to keep a steady bedtime and wake up routine so that it is easier to manage my symptoms.

Food

This has been a game changer for me to see improvements. It's not easy, because I love bread and sweets like most people do. I can now feel the difference if I eat something that doesn't work for my body. Occasionally I choose to eat the wrong things, but a smaller portion and not often seems to be the best approach to this for now, even though it may cause symptoms to be more pronounced.

Gluten

Gluten has an effect on my digestive system, and I am so much better when I eat gluten-free. I have also noticed that when I cave in and have food with gluten, I am in more pain. It really depends on what the food is and how long I end up not paying attention to this. This is very hard to do, because I am not allergic to gluten but I do have sensitivities. Once I was eating gluten-free for a while, I started noticing how I felt when I ate whatever I wanted. It takes moderation or a completely gluten-free diet for me to feel the best benefits on pain and fatigue.

Refined Sugars

I love desserts! In fact, the theme of our wedding was "All you need is love and dessert," as it was an early afternoon wedding. We had a full dessert buffet and the guests loved it! But all those refined sugars, *uuuugh*! Anyway, I have come to learn that refined sugars cause me much grief. I can tell when I have had too much, as my body is in more pain, the brain fog is worse, and I am more tired. It takes days to recover. It took me a while to see the pattern, but when we pay attention to the factors around us when our bodies are "talking" to us, we can begin to see the patterns.

New Sources of Joy

One of the things that helps is to find new sources of joy that help you to relax and rest. For me, this happens to be camping. We bought a used trailer, and this is a great way for me to recharge. The key is to make it less work, not more. Our trailer sits in our yard and we keep it packed and ready to go. The only thing we need to do is pick up a few groceries and we are off. This transient style of camping works better than being at one place. For one, it is less work because you just pull in and park, and, second, you get to explore new places. Another surprise form of relaxation for me was going hunting with my husband. I got all my certifications and licenses and started deer hunting annually with my husband. I tell you, sitting in the woods in the crisp fall is the most relaxing and peaceful holiday I have ever had. This is a great place to meditate, pray, and focus for me. I am conscious of having to be comfortable, so I ensure that I have some creature comforts with me, such as a comfortable camping chair and heated mitts and boots (you can buy little packets for both). I also do not stay out for long periods of time. Since mornings are my worst time, I tend to go for a short time in the afternoon. But this activity has been something I have come to look forward to because I know how I feel when I come home. I recently began to knit again, and I have found this to be a restful activity. Two years ago, I could not have done this because my cognitive abilities would not have allowed me to do so. I am also back to reading for pleasure. At one point, I could not read a paragraph and comprehend it. Last summer I started to read again and over time couldn't believe how quickly I was able to bring this back. It just took time and ensuring I had the rest that was essential to recharge my batteries. Another activity that has become relaxing for me is landscape painting. It was something I had wanted to do but never took the time. I am still looking for activities and new sources of joy, but I am happy to have a few to focus on now and this keeps me feeling positive for having a fulfilling life living with fibromyalgia and depression.

Measuring Progress and Checking In

This is crucial to being able to make strides in improvement. If you're like me and most people with fibromyalgia, you have a type A personality. You want to feel better now and are not used to having to take extended amounts of time to accomplish things. This is one of those things you need to allow yourself to be patient with. If you are, I promise you will start to see improvement and then more improvement comes sooner. I can help you check in with yourself and measure progress, especially when you think you are not improving. It's a big balancing act of self-care, taking baby steps, and learning to put you first.

Something else that happened for me to see a change for the better was in my ability to read. I have been a pleasure reader for many years now, and it was always a great way to de-stress at the end of a day to relax and fall asleep. But during the worst years of illness I lost the ability to do this. I tried so many times but would give up when I couldn't remember what I had read on a page or even in just one paragraph. I couldn't remember day-to-day what I was trying to read. I gave up on this. But, when this started to improve, I knew this was a good sign. In the beginning I had to reread paragraphs and sometimes pages from the night before to recall the storyline, but I was starting to be able to stay with it and comprehend what I was reading. It sounds strange because I did so much research on my illness, but I think that was my brain's way of keeping me focused to find a way to be well. Reading became enjoyable again, and when I continued to persevere, it became easier and easier until I was back to reading novels. My mother even commented on how fast I was now going through books again. This was an amazing feeling and a really good indicator of progress for me and it may be for you as well.

Stress

This is a big one. Many sources talk about the effect of stress and the diagnosis of fibromyalgia. Long-term chronic stress is, and can be, a catalyst to triggering fibromyalgia. There are also sources that point to one traumatic event that triggers fibromyalgia. I could not figure out why this all happened to me until I learned the possible triggers of fibromyalgia and major depression. Once I did, I was able to pinpoint why and the moment life changed for me. I truly believe it could have been avoided had I realized what the long-term stress was doing to me. I was always able to handle and push through, but this one experience in the workplace traumatized me and I ended up sick and off work. My psychiatrist described what I had gone through as having an emotional stroke. My brain was working differently and had been hurt. I needed medication and therapy to help it get better. He also said that, like a stroke, you may not fully recover, but you can certainly make great improvements to have a satisfying and joy-filled life. I proved this could be done, and you can do it, too. I can help you with this so that you do not have to take as long as it took me to feel improvements, and you can work toward your goal of working again.

Weather

Many people are affected by changes in weather. My daughter's knees ache when it's going to rain, and I know many people who describe similar issues. Fibromyalgia is greatly affected by weather. This is a major trigger for me. My chiropractor will even see more of his fibromyalgia patients when the weather systems change. He's able to know how I'm feeling because of how many fibromyalgia patients he will see in certain weather conditions. I am still working on figuring this one out and trying to predetermine based on forecasts how I might feel or when I might have a flare-up. I know for sure when there are big swings with pressure systems, from high to low or low to high, my muscles are in a lot of pain and I have more fatigue for a day or two leading up to the change. Learning to roll with this is a challenge but can be managed. Accepting it is half the battle. Learning to let go, listen to your body, rest, and do the things that make you feel better is important. That may include a massage, getting in a hot bath or hot tub, an additional chiropractor adjustment, and more rest than usual.

This is essential for you to bounce back so you can do things you want to do.

Church/Faith

I bring this up here because, for me, this was the final piece to the puzzle. From the time I was a young child I remember my mom taking us to church, and I did this with my children, too. For a while I had gotten away from it and had been really missing it, or rather God was calling me back. So we started going to church again about six months ago. For me, this was the missing link to further improvement. It brought me together, so to speak, mind, body, and spirit. I know this part will continue to grow and I have to thank God for the challenges I have been put through, especially this one. If not for these challenges, I would not be here writing this book to be able to help you manage your symptoms and get back to the career you love and thought you had to give up. It seems like such a simple thing, but there is so much negativity around being a Christian today and attending church is has become difficult for many. No matter what your faith, I believe this will be a major part of your final step to feeling better and fulfilling God's purpose He has in mind for you.

Chapter 10:

WOW! I Think I'm Ready to Work Again!

Myth: *You will never work again.*

Fact: *Managing symptoms improves the quality of your life so you can work and enjoy life again.*

I can still remember when I began to think that maybe there was a chance I could go back to teaching again. The thought actually surprised me, and I wasn't sure I could actually trust what I was feeling. I talked to my psychiatrist about this and she said to take it very slow. I was continuing to follow her advice because she was responsible for getting me to where I was at that point. I couldn't believe I was thinking about work again in a positive light. This didn't mean that I was better, it meant that I had improved that much and that the medication was starting to work on the chemical imbalances in my brain. It boggles my mind that our society is so empathetic when people have physical illnesses and that any treatment they seek out is seen as positive. While society has come a long way in thinking and acknowledging mental health it has not come far enough. Our brains are the CEOs for the rest of our bodies, but somehow there is a negative stigma when mental health issues and invisible illnesses present themselves. I experienced this firsthand, and this only added to the decline and persistent symptoms of my health. When I began to feel a positive change (thinking about teaching again), it didn't mean that I was better. It meant that we had finally found a medication mix that was beginning to treat the depression. It did not mean the depression was gone, as that is something I will have to manage the rest of my life. But it did give me hope. At first it scared me, because what if the feeling didn't last? This was September of 2017, and I was thinking about returning to work when the second semester started in February of 2018. I knew there was no way to go full time yet and my doctor, quite frankly, was keeping me from making a big mistake and taking on too much, too fast. So, we began to plan for my return around how the depression was and how I was managing the fibromyalgia symptoms. At this point I was still only able to manage about 1,200 steps daily before being exhausted. But I was gradually working on adding in more. This was difficult to do, as I wanted to go too quickly but from experience of setting myself back, I knew I had to take it slowly and still pace myself.

My doctor and I created a return to work plan so that I could start teaching one class second semester and it could only be in the afternoon, as mornings were still difficult for me. So, in December, two months before second semester began, I volunteered my time so that I could work up to teaching one class. To the average well person this might sound too simple, but it was the only way to ensure I would not be set back too hard. I started with a couple of days (one class) the first couple of weeks and gradually increased to be able to go in every day for the one class. I was only doing this by shadowing another teacher. It kept the stress level low for me and allowed me to get back into the routine and around students again. Working with the wellness and disability management officer in the human resources department was, and still is, a very positive experience for me. This was a new position to our school board and she played a key role in making my return to work experience an easier transition and a positive one. She was someone who had empathy for what I was dealing with and had my best interests in mind while bridging me back to the classroom. Her support continues to play a significant part in my ongoing transition back to full-time employment in the job I love.

I was also continuing my counselling sessions with a resident psychiatrist, and this was necessary to work through the anger and bitterness I still was holding from the traumatic experience at work that took me off work. This was also essential to my recovery and moving forward. Both he and my regular psychiatrist collaborated on my path back to wellness.

In order to get back to work it is essential to work with your doctor, do research, and decide what accommodations you will need in order to return to work. These are your human rights and I suggest that you check the laws in your area to ensure you get the support you need. In addition to only teaching one class, I needed to minimize the number of steps I would be taking in one day. The school I work in is large, so my classroom ended up being upstairs; however, it was at the top of the stairs from the entrance I took into the school. I was also able to park near that entrance. My office was near the classroom I was teaching in. This was essential for me not to burn out my energy and be unable to do my job, as managing a classroom full of teenagers can be exhausting even for someone who is well. I also needed physical support, and this was accommodated with the type of chair I got for my classroom and office. Working with the wellness officer, we were able to get the perfect chair to support me when I needed to work at my desk and when I needed to take a break from standing and walking around the classroom too much. To balance this, I purchased the same chair for my office at home. This was another game changer for me. It was just a chair, but I know that it has and continues to be the support I need to do my work. My pain has been reduced by having a proper office chair for my needs. I also received a special light that simulates exposure to the sun. I use this daily in the morning to help with the symptoms of depression.

Another key accommodation was the distance I could drive to work. Any driving over thirty minutes did, and does, exhaust me, so teaching at a school further away than that was not going to work. This continues to work for me, and when I do have to make the trek to see my doctor and have to drive over thirty minutes, I am worn out and need to rest. Teaching is exhausting enough for me, but having to make a longer commute to and from work would not be beneficial and would greatly affect my ability to do my job well.

Returning to work after four plus years was difficult because I was returning to a different school, yet again. While I only knew a few people, I wasn't close to anyone because I had been off for so long. I felt brand new again and that was difficult to cope with. I was fortunate to get two very supportive coworkers to shadow for my gradual return. I don't know how I could have done it without their support. I am grateful for all they did to help make a difficult situation a positive one so I could focus on doing what I love.

By the time second semester rolled around, I felt ready to take on a class of my own. This was very intimidating, and I was so nervous. I would be teaching a subject I had taught before, so this helped with preparation. I ended up with a terrific group of students (twenty-eight in total), and they made my return to the classroom the best experience possible. Again, I was grateful that it turned out this way.

The key to returning to work is support. Support from both the employer and at home. I had made significant improvements in my health but knew I was going to need to learn to manage all my symptoms again so that I could do my job and continue to improve with the goal of teaching full time again. I was nervous, but that was soon put at ease as the wellness and disability management officer was wonderful to work with and completely understood my needs. She made me feel like I was welcome once again and that she was there to support my return to work for whatever I needed. I cannot emphasize how important this was to my successful return to work and also my ongoing success to continue to work. Seek out the people in your workplace who will get you the support you need and be there for you when you need to check in. All of those same issues that put you off work could very well still be there, and when you have someone who is on your side it's a great feeling. I knew I could check in with her when I needed to.

I know in my heart you can do this. Without the knowledge I learned from becoming a fibromyalgia advisor, I would not have been able to make the improvements I did. I took all I learned and implemented a number of strategies that helped me to improve my health and be able to get back to the career I love so much and enjoy life again. I want this same goal for you as well. I know you miss your job and it is part of you, it is part of what defines the person you are, and is important for your mental well-being. I never thought for a second that I would be able to work again, let alone return to teaching. This was the most difficult thought that I struggled with daily. For me, returning to work, even to teach one class, was what ended up helping me to find joy again in my job. It was exhilarating to feel this again and is what kept me moving forward to manage my symptoms. I gradually began to feel comfortable in my surroundings. It took time for me to be able to expand the number of coworkers that I communicated with, so at first I just came in, taught the class, and then left when I had prepared the next day's lesson. As time went on this improved greatly, and I began to feel like part of the team. I met with the wellness advisor regularly and felt that she had my best interests at heart and wanted to see me thrive in my job again.

After that first semester ended, summer came and my doctor and I made the decision that I could try to add another class to my teaching schedule. The key to this working was only scheduling my classes for afternoons. I still deal with brain fog, stiffness, and pain in the mornings.

I am now on track to add back in my last class to return to full time, but I know I need to have it scheduled for late morning and not have the first period of the day. My hope and goal at this point is to return to full time this fall, 2019.

Strategies list to keep in mind:

- Partner with your doctor and other health care providers.
- Continue to take medication as necessary. Don't listen to the stigma around meds. Trust your body and your doctor.
- Do your own research to find accommodations that you know will work for you and your body.
- Have an advocate at work who you work with and who positively supports your return

- Get any physical accommodations you need to support your body.
- Be kind to yourself and don't push too hard.
- Acknowledge that you are vulnerable and it could be easy to return to old habits
- Incorporate into your routine activities to reduce stress and pain, such as yoga, meditation, and relaxation/rest. Make this a must in your schedule.
- Stop beating yourself up when you don't think you've done enough. You have come a long way and still have time to make more improvements.
- Listen to your body and your gut. When it's time to rest, it's time to rest!

Chapter 11:

Why Am I Having a Bad Day Again?

Myth: *You can think yourself better.*

Fact: *Learning to listen to your body and discovering what strategies work best for you helps to minimize symptoms, and you will recover quicker when they return.*

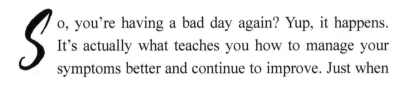o, you're having a bad day again? Yup, it happens. It's actually what teaches you how to manage your symptoms better and continue to improve. Just when

you think you're on your way to better, *boom,* it hits again. I actually started calling it hitting the wall, because that is what it felt like. It was not a gradual feeling, either. I knew I was feeling a bit tired and would continue what I was doing but didn't realize that my recharged battery was going to crash or hit the wall. When this happens, it doesn't matter what you're doing because you need to immediately lie down and rest. Some, even many, might think, "Really, is it that bad?" Oh, trust me, it is. Only my closest family and friends ever see this, because it usually happens at home after I've done too much in that day and continued to do more at home. Or after a long week when I've continued to do stuff on the weekend. It can also strike after you've had a great day and then you think you can continue, and that is when you hit the wall.

In writing this chapter, I realize I don't hit that wall nearly as much anymore. I've learned to listen to my body cues and not care what people think because I know how I feel. This is not something you can just push through and keep going. I know what that is because that is what I always did it to accomplish anything. This is so much different, and it has total control over what you are able to do. If you don't take forced rest, your symptoms will get worse again and recovery takes even longer. I know, because I've done it.

One example happened last September on the first professional activity day we had. Our principal had planned a great day of team building and collaboration at an outdoor education centre. While mornings are really tough for me, I planned all week so that I could try to attend this. I knew I would have the weekend to recover if any symptoms were made worse. But I was not prepared for how bad I was going to feel. I attended and really enjoyed the activities but ended up staying too long and sitting at picnic tables. Really, it was the perfect storm of doing the wrong things for my body. By Monday I had to take a sick day and it took me two weeks to get my symptoms back on track and feel well again. That was a huge learning curve. People just don't understand the invisibleness of this illness and the effects it has. Moving forward, I knew I would have to just switch my day and attend the morning so I could rest in the afternoon. This has been a good plan for me. It really depends on what the day is going to look like and what we are doing, and then I can plan how to structure my day for optimum benefit to me.

You will face challenges again. This is hard work, but don't be discouraged because it takes time to climb this mountain and pacing yourself is essential. Having someone who's been there in your corner to help with those daily challenges and set goals to manage them is a really good idea. Before you even realize it, you can reflect and begin to see progress. I am now at a much better place with my health and have had a significant increase in my abilities. I have gotten so tuned in to how I feel I can usually guess how many steps I've taken. I am careful to not go over too much because that is when my energy depletes while fatigue and pain increase. I first used my phone to track steps but then got a fitness tracker to monitor more closely. This is a great tool to help you manage so that you don't overdo it and you can prepare yourself to get home and rest before you burn out your batteries on any given day. Do I ever overdo it now? Yes, but I choose when it is something I really, really want to do and understand the effects it will have on my body. It takes planning for though, and that must be done before and after the event or whatever you plan on doing. As I learned in my coaching course, these times are referred to as flare-worthy.

I want you to understand that you can't think yourself better. You may hear people say "It's all in your head, positive thoughts produce positive results," but this just doesn't work – at least, for me it didn't – and I don't know anyone with fibromyalgia who has been able to do that. Just like major depression, it takes medication, food changes, lifestyle changes, and strategies to manage symptoms and flare-ups. This is not all in your head. Thankfully, research continues to dispel this myth. While strides have been made in understanding fibromyalgia, fatigue, chronic pain, depression, and anxiety, further research is necessary to change the way insurance companies, doctors, and people in general view these chronic illnesses.

Once you have more good days than bad you will begin to identify triggers to flare-ups. As I described before, the trigger on the PA day for me was just overdoing it for too long in the day and not sitting on a proper chair to avoid pain. There are many triggers to having flare-ups and you will discover triggers that will be different to someone else. At times you may not even know what caused the flare-up and you will be forced to put yourself as the priority and manage your symptoms. The sooner you jump on doing the right things, such as rest and pain management, the sooner you will be back to feeling good again. This is hard, as it can easily affect your mood and you can spiral into being very down and feeling negative. That's normal, and once you're able to identify and strategize for such times you'll feel better about choosing what and when to do things. Making a list of what your priorities are is essential. Mine include spending time with my husband – times for relaxation including vacations that don't cause me to overdo it – and getting back to my dream career. Living with constant fatigue and pain shouldn't be tolerated by health-care practitioners. It takes a combination of modalities to manage fibromyalgia and major depression symptoms so that you can live life to your fullest and be happy. You need to be the CEO of your health and advocate for what you need. Do not underestimate this and don't settle for anything less than wellness, whatever that means for you.

For the most part, I manage the brain fog and pain as it ebbs and flows so that I can now work. My biggest issue is still fatigue. I never feel refreshed in the morning. This is something that my doctor and I are working on solving through another sleep analysis to see what is going on and if changes can be made to the CPAP machine settings to improve this. I sure hope so, as it is one of the hardest things to accept because I was always so active. Fibromyalgia is not a lazy person's illness and every career-minded individual I know with fibromyalgia are driven and achieve their goals, and more than likely have been dealing with too much long-term stress by rising to whatever challenge is placed in front of them, not knowing the negative impact it will/could have on their health and life in general. The difficulty is that no two people present the same way. While there are many similarities, there are so many differences that it challenges doctors to be able to make a diagnosis. Usually it involves a lot of testing and process of elimination to finally land on the fibromyalgia diagnosis. What works for you might not work for me and vice versa. Getting to know your body and paying attention to your surroundings is really important in how you manage your symptoms.

Two other things that will cause me to not feel as well or my symptoms to worsen are changes in stress levels and physical activity changes. I believe stress is one of the worst, if not *the* worst thing to take me down. In the past, good stress was a motivator for me and it is a really good thing in our lives in order to achieve our goals and grow as people. But regardless of good or bad stress, both will and can cause symptoms to worsen. Bad stress is a nightmare for me and can take me out for days on end. The best thing for me to do is avoid situations and people who cause me the most stress. This has been a challenge, but I am now able to confidently prioritize my health and say no when necessary, especially if I know it will make my symptoms flare.

All my life I loved to be active with things such as bike riding, walking, skiing, and being outside. I have had to alter how and if I include these in my life. I have learned to include things like yoga, meditation, and camping so that I relax more and reduce any stress that may be affecting my health. Camping has been a great activity to add in. It gives me time to relax and enjoy being outdoors, and it has given my husband the opportunity to also learn to relax. While I can't walk the distances I once did or at the same pace, I have been able to improve the number of steps I take, and I have hope that in the future I can do more.

The challenges of living with fibromyalgia and major depression are many, and at one point I didn't think my quality of life would ever improve. I'm sure that is where you're at and one of the reasons you are reading this now. It took me too long to figure things out and get to where I am. While I continue to face obstacles, they no longer make me feel that I am a failure. They encourage me to learn and to overcome them as best I can for my body so I can achieve the things I want to achieve, like returning to my teaching career.

Chapter 12:

Loving the New Me!

Myth: *Fibromyalgia is a career killer!*

Fact: *You can manage fibromyalgia symptoms and enjoy your life and career again.*

At the beginning of this book, you wanted to manage your fibromyalgia symptoms so that you could get back to the life and career you love. You wanted to feel you had a purpose again, but first you needed to somehow manage the pain, fatigue, and lack of energy that comes along with fibromyalgia. This illness can be a lonely one to navigate and find relief from, but there are many people diagnosed every year. It is a problem in our society. There are many myths in our society around fibromyalgia and I have done my best to try and dispel some of those myths for you in this book.

You learned how to reflect and identify the stress and/or situations that may have caused you to crash with illness and the importance of using good resources to educate yourself and to give you the support you need so you can focus on improving your symptoms.

I shared my struggle and the uphill battle that took me far too long to make progress. While my own doctors have said that very few go from where I was to where I am now, I believe it was because I self-advocated to get the help I needed. I kept an open mind and tried many, many different approaches to find and sustain feeling better. I also believe anyone can do it!

You learned to begin understanding your symptoms and that your pain and fatigue are real. You learned that rest is an integral part to starting to feel well. By now you also know that the feeling of loneliness is real due to the nature of the invisible symptoms you have but you do not have to feel that way. There are strategies and things to keep in mind so you don't face this alone.

You've learned that it's okay to need help and that it is essential for you to get the support you need with all of the day-to-day stuff so you can avoid feeling overwhelmed and down on yourself.

There is so much stuff out there on our health and wellness these days that it's hard to decide who to listen to and how to filter and flesh out what you need for you. I touched on many specialists, alternative practitioners, and therapies to help you begin your journey and see what works for you. I've given you a practical approach to start your journey back to the career you are so missing. I did not include all of the science stuff and medical jargon. Honestly that was a lot for me to take in when I was at my worst.

I still research and read to continue to make progress, but I am at a much better place to be able to take in the information and help others. By no means do I spend a lot of time on this. When I began to take on my health and tackle both depression and fibromyalgia, I needed simple steps, because cognitively I was not in a good place to digest too much information. I started with what I believed to be my biggest symptom and went from there. It was only then that I could start to see the hope and possibility that I would return to work. I love guiding and teaching teenagers and it all begins with baby steps for them to see their potential. I took this philosophy and used it to build on my own progress in managing my symptoms.

You learned to watch for the signs of starting to improve, measuring success, and finding new sources of joy, and that it is possible to begin to feel like you are going to return to the job you love. I've included obstacles you may face when having a bad day again, but this will help you to be prepared when they do strike. You will understand it will be short-term and that you can recover more easily because you have the tools and knowledge to do so.

My wish for you is that you do not have to give up a career or job and life you love just because you have fibromyalgia. Fibromyalgia is not a career killer like you and I once thought! By now I hope you're thinking that you know it's possible to get back to work and manage your symptoms. It may be something you think you can accomplish on your own. However, I believe one of the best ways to achieve your full potential with all of the challenges you face with fibromyalgia is having a coach/advisor so that you can have someone to talk to and to guide you as you learn to function in your "new" body. You will no doubt get there faster than I did trying to do it on my own. I became a fibromyalgia advisor to help myself, but in doing so have realized I need and want to help others. While I have been back at my teaching job for over a year now and loving it, I have this calling of sorts to help others. I never want to see anyone go through the pain and agony I have. It almost finished me. So when I was given the opportunity to help myself so that I may be able to help others, I took it. I love teaching and I look at this as a new teaching opportunity to make a bigger difference in this world. I will be your partner on your journey to advocate for your health, manage your symptoms, return to the job you love in less time than it took me, and be less likely to fall into your old patterns again. I want you to love your new self and find your joy in conquering fibromyalgia.

Thank you for staying with me on this journey! Now, let's get you get back to the career you love!

Acknowledgments

Thank you to David Hancock and the Morgan James Publishing team for helping me bring this book to print.

Tami Stackelhouse: I would be remiss if I did not acknowledge Tami for all of her support and for teaching me to become a fibromyalgia advisor. Even though I was in a very bad place, Tami not only took the time to care but saw something in me that I did not see for myself. She is the reason I even considered writing a book, introducing me to Angela and the Author Incubator team. Tami, I look forward to our paths intersecting again and doing great things together.

To the Author Incubator team: Special thanks again to Angela Lauria, CEO and founder of The Author Incubator, for believing in me and my message. I still can't believe you chose me! To my developmental editor, Mehrina, and managing editor, Bethany, thanks for making the process seamless and easy. Many more thanks to everyone else at TAI, but especially Cheyenne and Ramses for always being there for us authors in training. Do you two ever sleep?

Amanda Allison: Where do I even begin to thank you for your friendship? You never gave up on me; in fact, your calls, texts or emails always came at just the right time when I needed it most. I will be forever grateful to you and will always be here for you. You will be the first employee I hire!

Darrell: You are the best husband, and I feel blessed to be your wife. Thank you for your unconditional love and support. You've been there for me in some of the most difficult struggles of my life and for that I am truly grateful. You know how very much you mean to me, and to be able to acknowledge it in this book is extra special. Consider this my rooftop! A friendship that spans thirty plus years to finally recognizing how much we really love each other was the best gift! I am grateful for everything our life was, is, and will be. There's no other I'd rather be on this journey with than you. I love you! XO

God: Last but certainly not least, I have to thank God for the many blessings in my life. I would not be where I am today without my faith and understanding that the most difficult challenges we face are all part of a bigger picture and plan that God has for us. When we truly believe, have faith and trust in God to put in front of us what we are meant to do, only then is it possible to accomplish something that is more amazing that you could dream of.

Thank You

I sincerely want to thank you for purchasing and taking the time to read my book. It was written for you! I felt that my struggle and challenges with fibromyalgia and depression had to be shared so that I can help others and make a positive difference in their lives. I never want to see anyone take as long as I did to get back to the things they love, especially their career. This is not the end for you either!

If you are serious and ready to have someone guide and support you through your own improvement journey I would love to talk with you. Please reach out to me by email at karen@karenbrinklow.ca. At the end of our chat you will be able to make a clear decision about working together. You are one step closer to managing your symptoms. It's time for you to feel better so you can enjoy life again. You may even want return to the job you love. I can't wait to help you get there. Together we can overcome anything!

Karen

About the Author

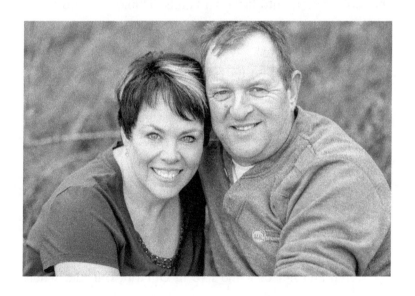

*K*aren Brinklow is a high school teacher and the first Certified Fibromyalgia Advisor in Canada. She helps successful professional women manage their fibromyalgia symptoms so they can focus on the career and life they love.

Karen became a teacher at age forty-one, after a career in business and sales. A teaching career was a dream come true, and she was thrilled when she was hired full time to build a business program in a local high school. About seven years into her career she was experiencing debilitating fatigue and pain, lack of energy, and profound feelings of sadness. Reluctantly, she had to take sick leave. After a few years on sick leave she became so frustrated with not feeling better she took matters into her own hands. Thinking she'd never be able to work again, she just wanted some relief from her symptoms. Karen says she can now look at this difficult time and diagnosis with gratitude, because she is now able to help others so they don't have to take as long to get back to the careers they love and to live their best life possible!

Karen loves the outdoors and especially taking time to relax camping. She loves the time she gets to take for self-care so she can be her best self for family and those who are needing her help. Karen returned to the teaching career she loves, but knew she had to help other professional women with similar problems.

Karen and her husband live in Ontario, Canada, where they enjoy country living, travel, and time with family.

CPSIA information can be obtained
at www.ICGtesting.com
Printed in the USA
JSHW020258210323
39183JS00003BC/590